PRINCIPLES OF PHOTOGRAPHY IN FACIAL PLASTIC SURGERY

Published Volumes

Proportions of the Aesthetic Face
Powell and Humphreys

Facial Reconstruction with Local and Regional Flaps
Becker

Rhinoplasty: Emphasizing the External Approach
Anderson and Ries

Surgery of the Mandible
Bailey and Holt

Lasers in Skin Disease
Wheeland

Dermabrasion and Chemical Peel
McCollough and Langsdon

Free Flap Reconstruction of the Head and Neck
Panje and Moran

Cosmetic Surgery of the Asian Face
McCurdy

Surgery of the Lip
Calhoun and Stiernberg

American Academy of Facial Plastic and Reconstructive Surgery

Series Editor: Charles M. Stiernberg, M.D.

PRINCIPLES OF PHOTOGRAPHY IN FACIAL PLASTIC SURGERY

M. Eugene Tardy, M.D., F.A.C.S.
Director of Facial Plastic Surgery
Department of Otolaryngology -
Head and Neck Surgery
University of Illinois Medical Center
Chicago, Illinois

and

Robert Brown, B.S.

with contributions to the medical photography by
Chet Childs, B.S.

1992
Thieme Medical Publishers, Inc., New York
Georg Thieme Verlag, Stuttgart • New York

Thieme Medical Publishers, Inc.
381 Park Avenue South
New York, New York 10016

Series sponsored by the educational committee of The American Academy of Facial Plastic and Reconstructive Surgery

PRINCIPLES OF PHOTOGRAPHY IN FACIAL PLASTIC SURGERY
M. Eugene Tardy

Library of Congress Cataloging-in-Publication Data

Tardy, M. Eugene, 1934–
Principles of photography in facial plastic surgery / M. Eugene Tardy and Robert Bown ; with contributions to the medical photography by Chet Childs.
p. cm.—(American Academy of Facial Plastic and Reconstructive Surgery)
Includes bibliographical references and index.
ISBN 0-86577-148-0 (Thieme Medical Publishers).—ISBN 3-13-661301-5 (Georg Thieme Verlag)
1. Face—Surgery. 2. Surgery, Plastic. 3. Photography, Medical. I. Brown, Robert J. (Robert James), 1960– . II. Title. III. Series: The American Academy of Facial Plastic and Reconstructive Surgery (Series)
[DNLM: 1. Face—surgery. 2. Neck—surgery. 3. Photography. 4. Surgery, Plastic. WE 705 T183p]
RD119.5.F33T37 1992
617.5′20592—dc20
DNLM/DLC
for Library of Congress 91-36871
CIP

Important Note: Medicine is an ever-changing science. Research and clinical experience are continually broadening our knowledge, in particular our knowledge of proper treatment and drug therapy. Insofar as this book mentions any dosage or application, readers may rest assured that the authors, editor and publishers have made every effort to ensure that such references are strictly in accordance with the state of knowledge at the time of production of the book. Nevertheless, every user is requested to carefully examine the manufacturers' leaflets accompanying each drug to check on his own responsibility whether the dosage schedules recommended therein or the contraindications stated by the manufacturers differ from the statements made in the present book. Such examination is particularly important with drugs which are either rarely used or have been newly released on the market.

Some of the product names, patents and registered designs referred to in this book are in fact registered trademarks or proprietary names even though specific reference to this fact is not always made in the text. Therefore, the appearance of a name without designation as proprietary is not to be construed as a representation by the publisher that it is in the public domain.

Printed in the United States of America

5 4 3 2 1

TMP ISBN 0-86577-148-0
GTV ISBN 3-13-661301-5

Contents

Preface

Standardized, uniform patient photographs are as essential to the head and neck surgeon as x-rays are to the orthopedist, audiograms to the otologist, and electrocardiograms to the cardiologist. Vivid, clear, and uniform pre- and postoperative photographs allow the surgeon to plan carefully and assess his work accurately. Excellent photographs assume major importance in the head and neck region, because the surgical outcome is highly visible for appreciation as well as criticism.

In all fields of modern medicine, *documentation* for accurate record-keeping, medicolegal purposes, and medical insurance coverage has been elevated to a level of importance surpassed only by uncompromising care of the patient. Standard and uniform photographs are no longer simply a pleasantly aesthetic adjunct to proper treatment, they are *mandatory.*

In a sense, all surgeons are teachers; only their audience varies. Whether teaching an international interspecialty audience of physicians, actively developing the thought processes of students and residents, or engaging in day-to-day enlightenment of patients concerned and cautious about their forthcoming surgery, well-taken and properly chosen photographs uniquely catalyze the teaching and communication process.

The self-teaching, self-confrontational aspects of long-term, standardized photographs are of special value to the surgeon. Sequential photographic comparison of the progressive phases of healing and postsurgical evolutionary changes provides the surgeon with an unparalleled, dispassionate assessment of his own skills and a clear record of how the dynamics of healing influence the "final outcome." No better method of continuing medical self-education exists.

Although gradually improving, the photographic skills of physicians are in need of constant evaluation and upgrading. Major presentations at medical meetings as well as articles in important journals too often contain completely unacceptable photographs and illustrations. In a sense, the surgeon's attention to photographic detail provides an important clue to his surgical skills and commitment to excellence, and he is commonly judged accordingly by his peers.

The purpose of this monograph is to document practical guidelines and techniques, in a simplified and straightforward manner, for creating standard and uniform photographs of consistently high quality. The approaches and recommendations contained herein are all in current use and, of equal importance, they work. Medical photography, like medicine, is both an art and a science. Like vintage recipes, however, results are usually best achieved by following the directions. Therefore, those just beginning careers in head and neck surgery are urged to follow these guidelines. As the skills involved in ensuring high-quality uniform and standard photographs are perfected, the development of new and tangential photographic methods will undoubtedly enhance the quality of enjoyment of your medical practice. The authors wish to acknowledge gratefully the following friends and colleagues whose teaching significantly influences much of what lies herein:

Jill Rudansky, whose highly professional editorial guidance in this and other publications has been invaluable; Mrs. Maria Ikenburg, RBP, who patiently but rigidly demonstrated (to any resident who would listen) the awesome but often subtle differences between a quality photograph and those of mediocre worth; Dr. Richard Buckingham, whose otologic photography remains unsurpassed to this day and who, in no uncertain terms, made me painfully aware of the futility of ever showing a poor slide; Dr. Paul H. Holinger, whose skill and infinite patience in securing that "one perfect photograph" are known to all otolaryngologists; and a large number of former residents and Fellows, who regularly challenge traditional approaches and delight in holding me accountable for any small (albeit temporary) fall from photographic grace.

M. Eugene Tardy Jr., M.D.

1 Elements of Ideal Medical Photographs

INTRODUCTION

In medical photography the recorded image should reflect as precisely and faithfully as possible exactly what is seen by the observer's eye. Unlike fashion, impressionistic, and artistic photography, for which intriguing and interesting illusions, shadows, and clever angles are intentionally created, medical photography for precise record-keeping should reveal only the exact, unimbellished image (Fig. 1). Although some artistic license can be exercised in the development of slide presentations and medical exhibits, the photographic images most often recorded and referred to—the pre- and postoperative photographs—should be absolutely standard and uniform in lighting, positioning, size, and color (Fig. 2). Within the limitations of varying film emulsions and processing variations, this goal is entirely possible and should be the aim of every surgeon engaged in any form of plastic and reconstructive surgery of the face and neck. By establishing and following certain standard, simple guidelines, uniformly excellent medical photographs can be achieved by anyone willing to be as careful about his photographic results as he surely is about his surgical results.

The question of whether or not the surgeon should become his own photographer is one for which there is no simple answer. For the most part, this monograph is written to provide some routine guidelines for the physician who wishes to improve the quality and uniformity of the photographs he utilizes. The surgeon is encouraged to become expert in the various aspects of medical photography, since special and unique additional information can be learned about the patient during photography being carried out by the surgeon. For example, it is constantly a source of amazement that defects, asymmetries, and irregularities, undetected or overlooked during even the most careful physical examination, are exposed blatantly when the patient is viewed through the camera lens. Accurate preoperative diagnosis and evaluation is thus facilitated and even enhanced.

Furthermore, important psychologic information is frequently revealed during the photographic sitting. The patient who is unable to strike and hold a recommended pose, who is fidgety, uncooperative, silly, and superficial, may indeed represent an extremely poor candidate for image-changing surgery. This vital information is likely to be unappreciated if the photographs are recorded by an office assistant or professional photographer.

More often than not, however, with the exception of large metropolitan and university or clinic settings, the only convenient photographer is the surgeon or his capable trained assistant. In the final analysis, it is the uncompromising standardized recording of uniform photographs from sitting to sitting that is important. Who performs this critical activity is purely a matter of personal interest, taste, and convenience.

Finally, situations arise on a regular basis in which the surgeon may want special, nonroutine views of patients with interesting problems in addition to the standardized series; unless this information is precisely conveyed to the photographer, the opportunity to record an important preoperative condition in a different and more instructive and revealing way may be lost forever.

An equally strong case may be made for assigning the responsibility for pre- and postoperative photographs to either a professional photographer or an interested office assistant. In an extremely busy surgical practice, assuming the responsibility for all photography imposes an additional, albeit minimal, burden on the surgeon's time. If professional assistance is available and convenient, there is much to recommend it.

OFFICE PHOTOGRAPHY

Taking and recording precise pre- and postoperative facial photographs should be an easy and pleasant photographic task for the surgeon, since a near foolproof system can be developed that requires only that the same protocol be followed from sitting to sitting, eliminating most variables. Since the lighting, background, camera-to-subject distance, and lens opening remain the same (these factors are dis-

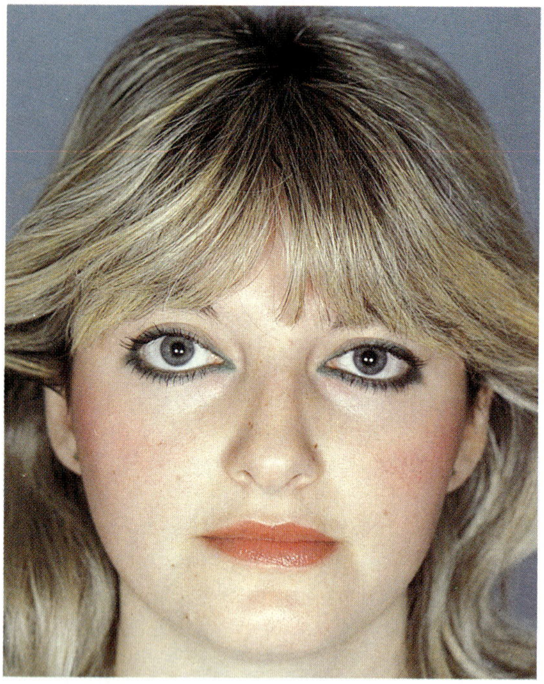

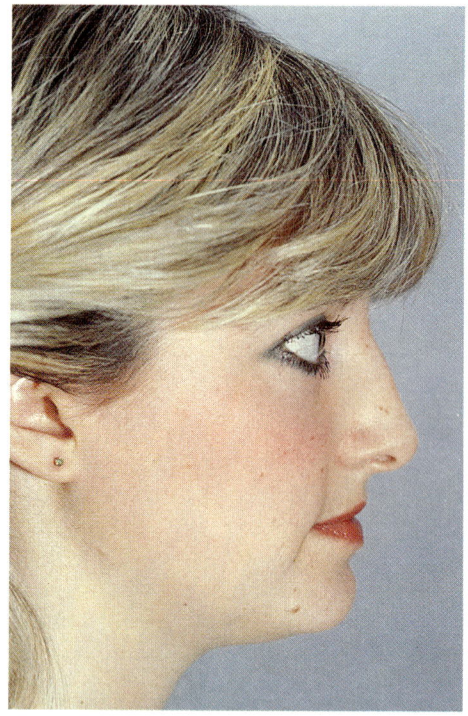

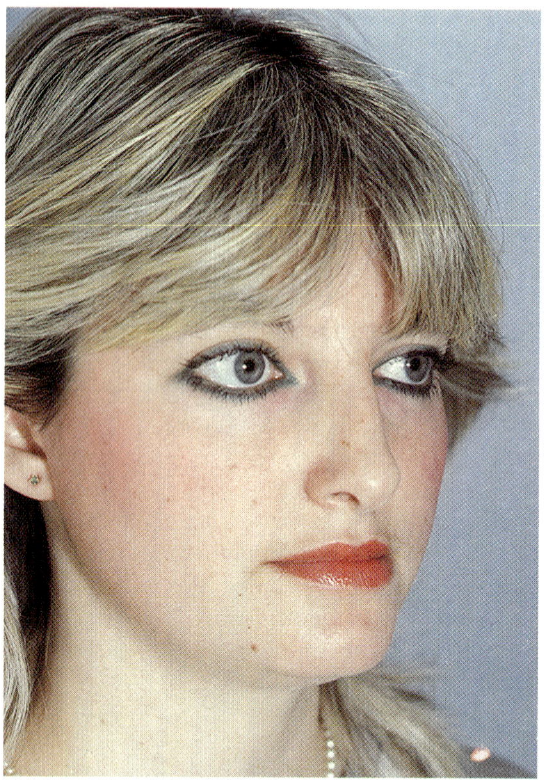

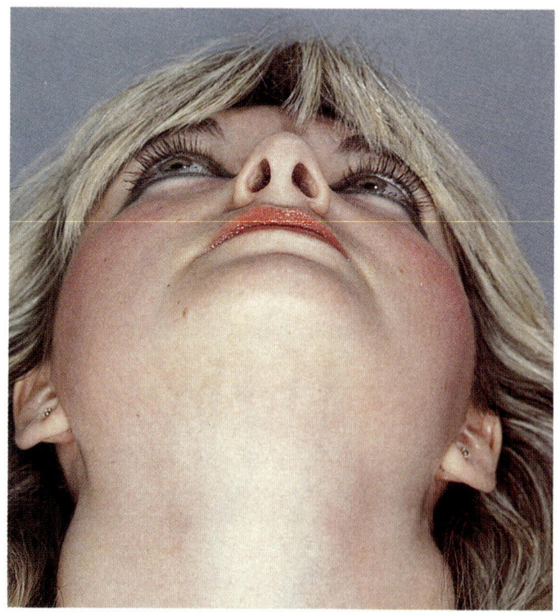

Figure 1. Ideal medical photographs should reveal as accurately as possible every unembellished detail of the patient's anatomy. Sufficient views should be recorded to allow accurate preoperative planning and postoperative assessment of long-term results.

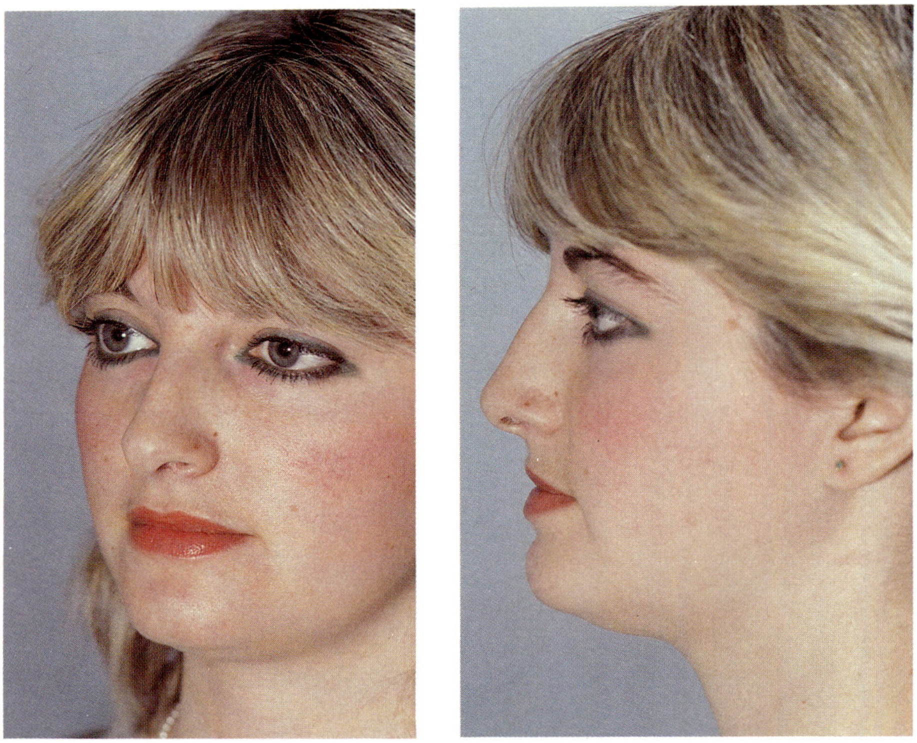

Figure 1. *(Continued)*

cussed later), the only requirement imposed on the photographer is to align the patient's face and head properly according to the positioning guidelines recommended.

Relatively strict rules should be applied to composition and positioning techniques, which are mandatory for uniform pre- and postoperative photographs. For accurate comparison of surgical results, both by an audience of learners as well as by the surgeon himself, precise reproducible positioning rules must be followed religiously. With the possible exception of aberrant lighting, *erratic positioning of the patient's head is the single most common transgression in facial photography.*

Patient Positioning

Not only is it unprofessional to project nonuniform pre- and postoperative photographs to a medical audience, it is misleading at best and deceptive at worst. Most photographic misrepresentation is clearly unintentional, but it is possible to enhance a postoperative photograph deliberately with altered positioning. Inaccurate patient positioning is the most common variable in standardized, uniform patient photographic documentation. Attention to small details can easily and quickly overcome this deficiency.

A seemingly ideal precise positioning device would simulate the common head-holder apparatus used by radiologists in obtaining accurate cephalometric radiographs. However, inconvenience and aesthetic distraction of such a device outweighs its effectiveness. Instead, the photographer must learn to rely on dead reckoning to create accurate and repeatable patient positions. Simple attention to detail, following universal guidelines, will allow appropriate spatial orientation of the head for uniformly accurate positioning.

The patient should be seated comfortably on a small rotating stool, at an elevation that will allow the feet to touch the floor, a stabilizing and security measure (Fig. 3). A small, short back on the stool is helpful to support and maintain erect posture, but it should not be high enough to be visible in the photograph (Fig. 4). Although the stool may be on rollers for ease and movement, it should be capable of stabilization in order that the camera-to-subject distance always remains constant, as does the distance from the patient to the light source.

Frankfort Horizontal Plane

The Frankfort horizontal plane is an imaginary line, parallel to the horizontal (Fig. 5a). This imaginary line runs from the cephalic margin of the tragus

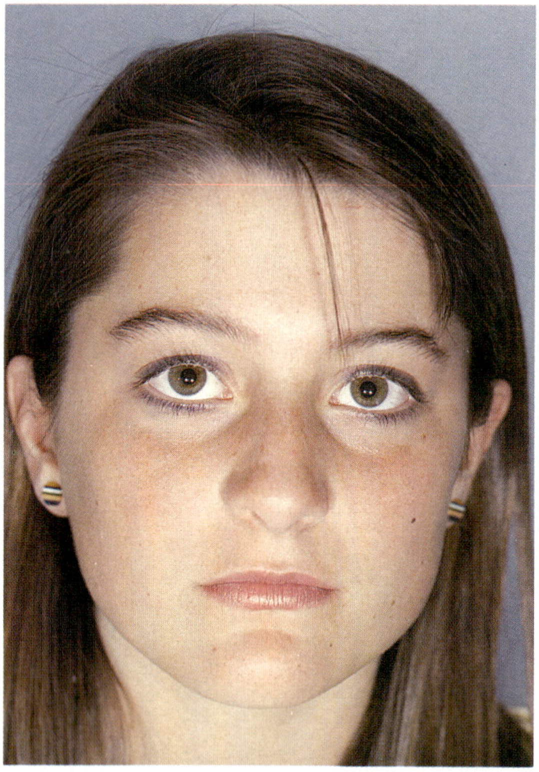

a

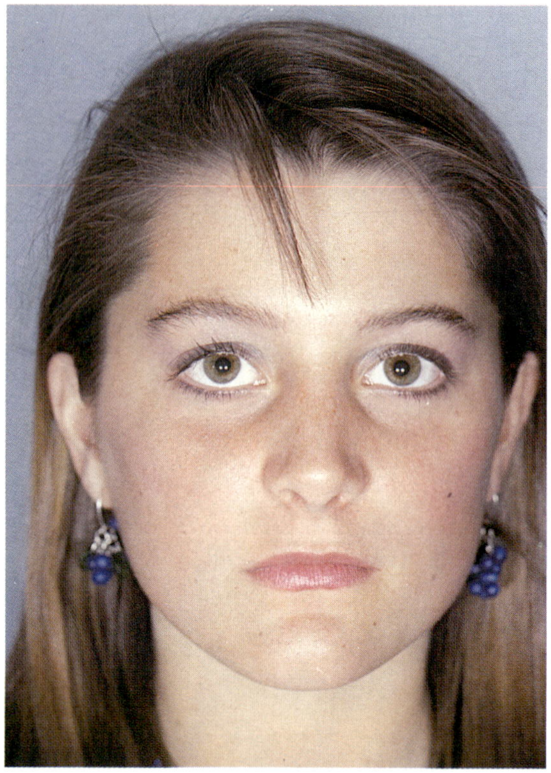

b

Figure 2. From sitting to sitting every effort should be expended to standardize lighting and positioning of the surgical patient, as in this series of photographs of a rhinoplasty patient recorded before surgery (A), at 1 month (B), and 1 year (C) after correction.

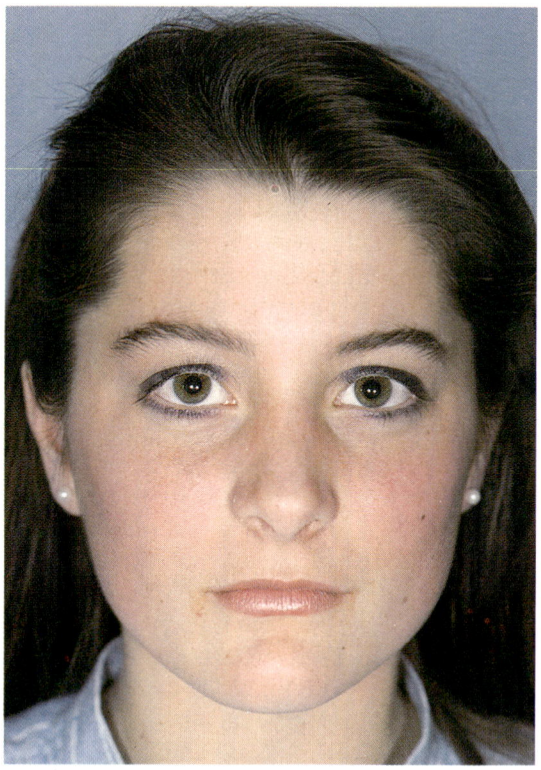

c

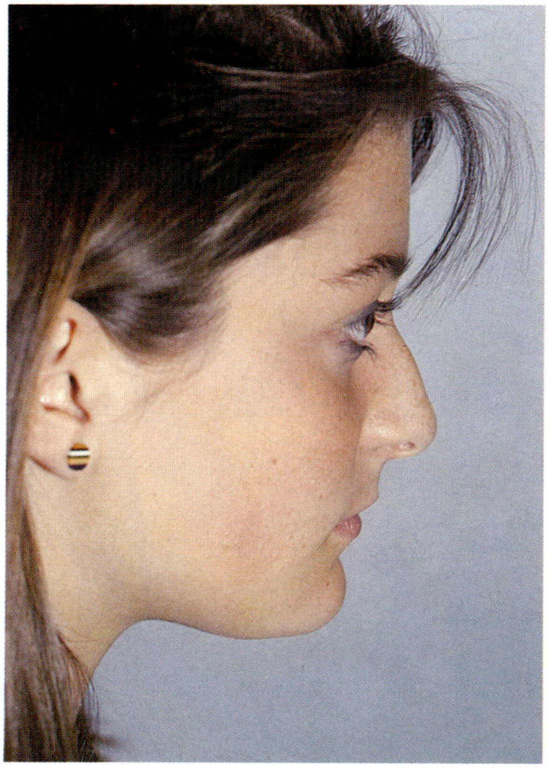
a

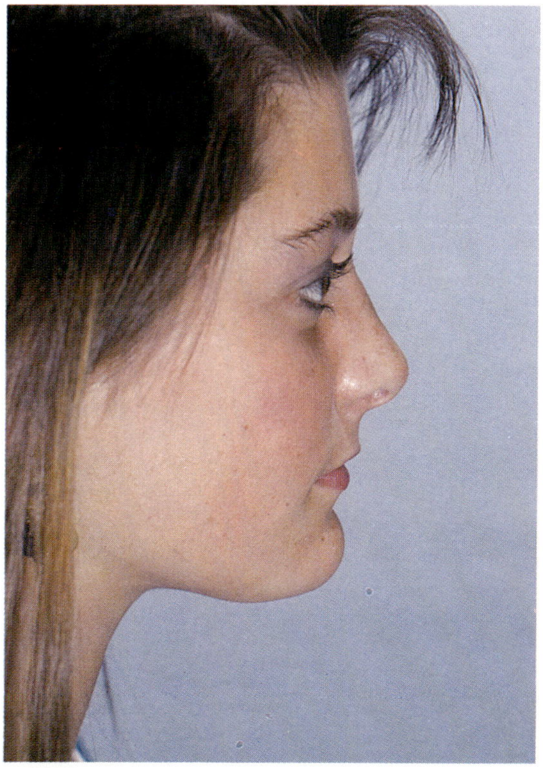
b

Figure 2. (*Continued*)

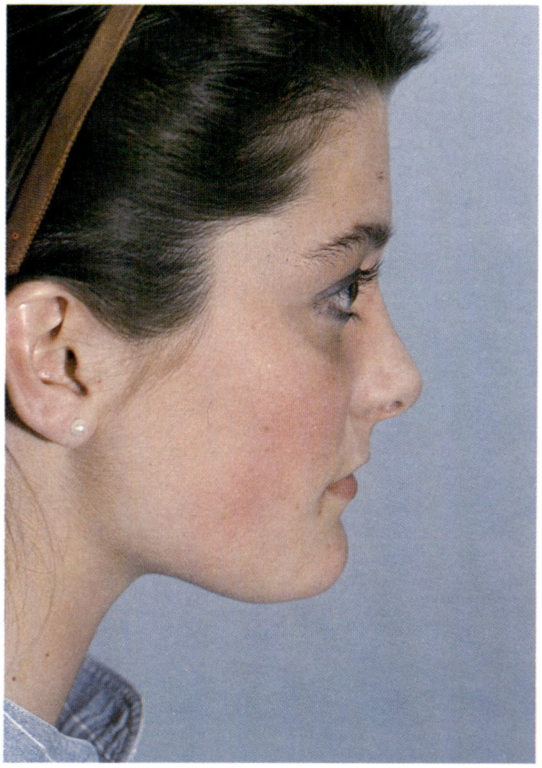
c

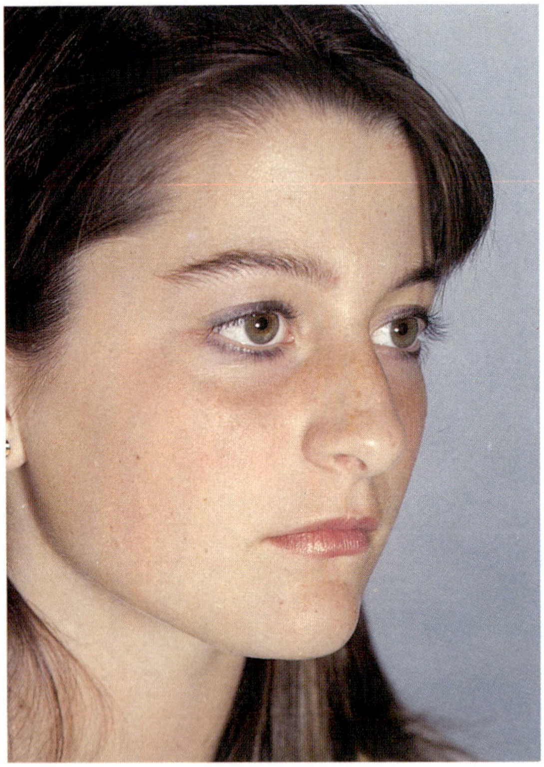
a

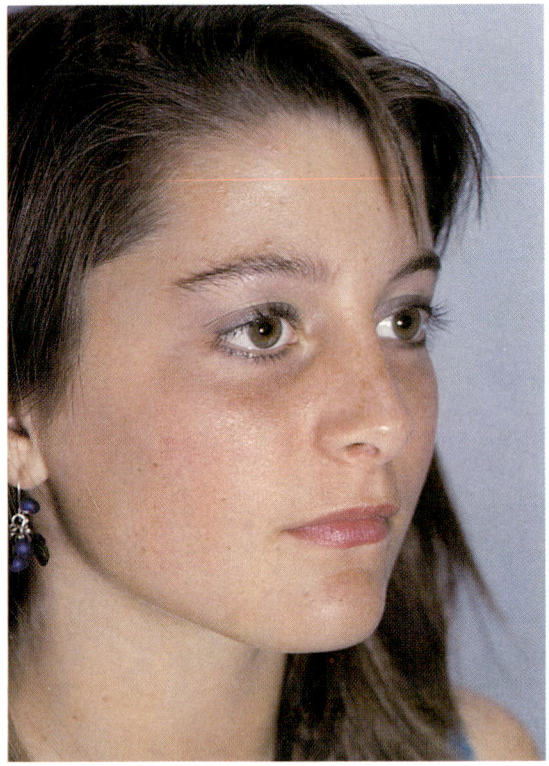
b

Figure 2. (*Continued*)

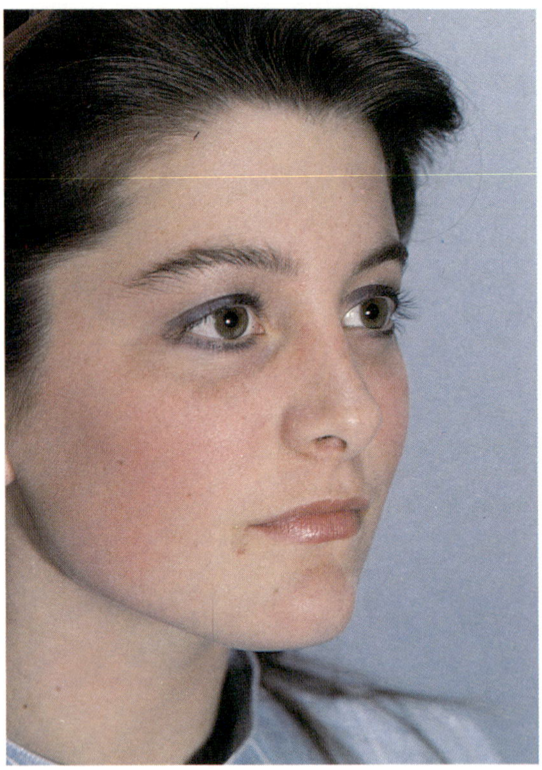
c

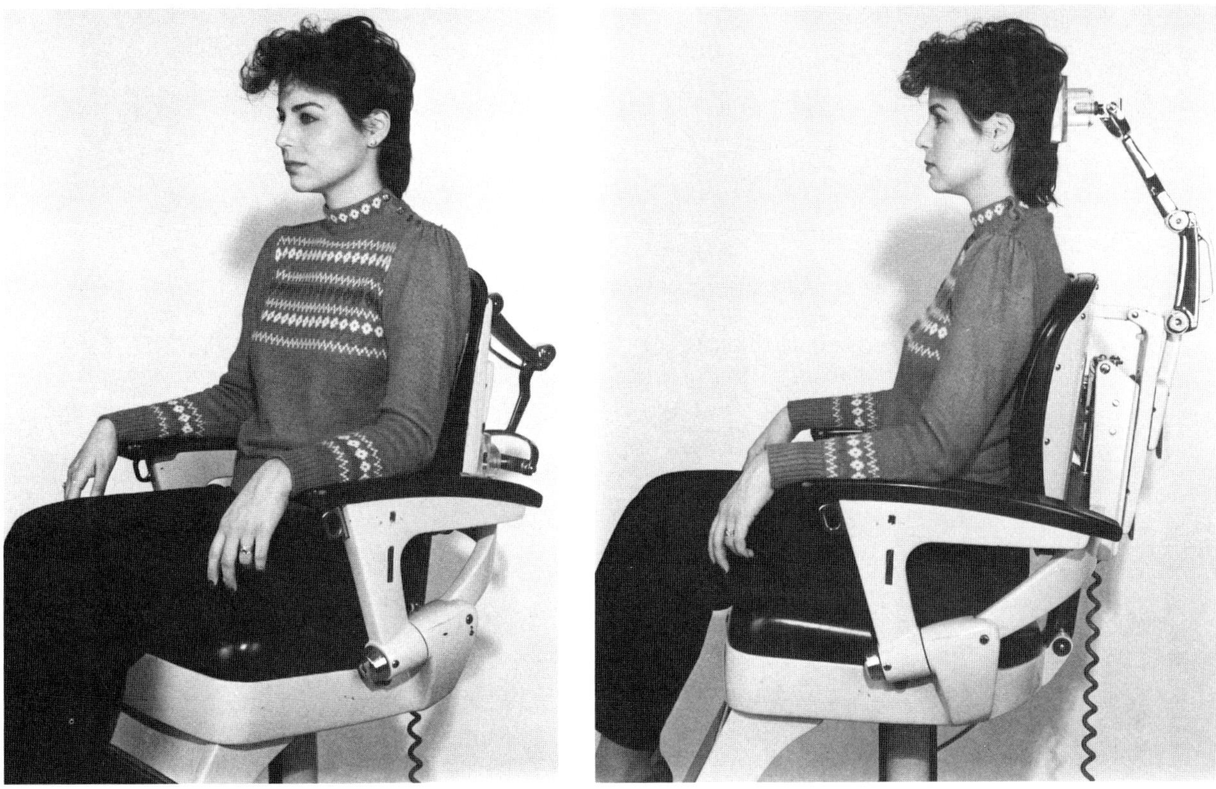

a b

Figure 3. **a,b,** A small rotating chair is ideal for patient positioning during photography, facilitating easy and rapid changes in desirable photographic views.

through the infraorbital rim (Fig. 5b and c) and must be the constant, stable positioning factor ever present in the photographer's eye and mind. As long as the patient is positioned with the Frankfort line parallel to the horizontal floor, the major variable factor in sequential positioning is made uniform and constant. The use of a grid-type viewing screen in the camera body is an immeasurable aid in proper patient alignment (Fig. 6a-e), but not all camera bodies accept interchangeable viewing screens. (This is a factor to consider when selecting a photographic system.)

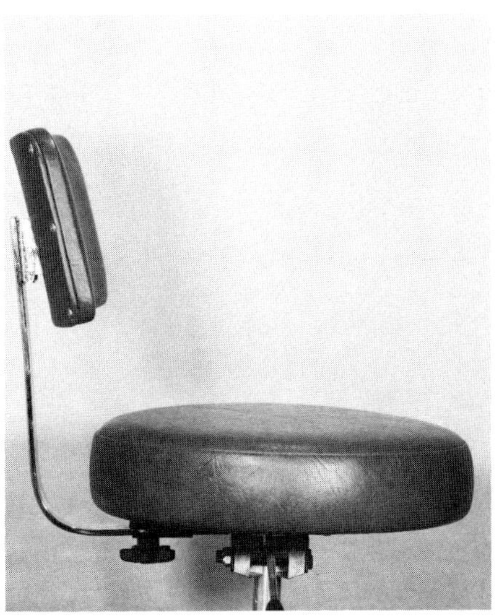

Figure 4. A short-backed stool aids in encouraging upright posture and stabilizes the patient during photography.

In reality, the Frankfort line is less suitable than it might be, since it is imaginary and on frontal view the top of the tragus may be difficult to visualize and one must often guess at the precise position of the infraorbital rim. Nonetheless, it is the most effective and reliable landmark available to the photographer and absolutely must be respected when framing facial images.

On frontal and base views, the midsagittal plane becomes a vital imaginary line (Fig. 6b and e). If, in positioning, the face deviates from this important plane, which is perpendicular to the horizontal, vital information may be lost, obscured, or misrepresented. Symmetric ears may look asymmetric, the nose may seem deviated, and eyes appear differently shaped.

The positioning guidelines provided by the Frankfort horizontal line and the midsagittal plane must be conscientiously respected by the surgeon-photographer. Frontal, lateral, oblique, and nasal base

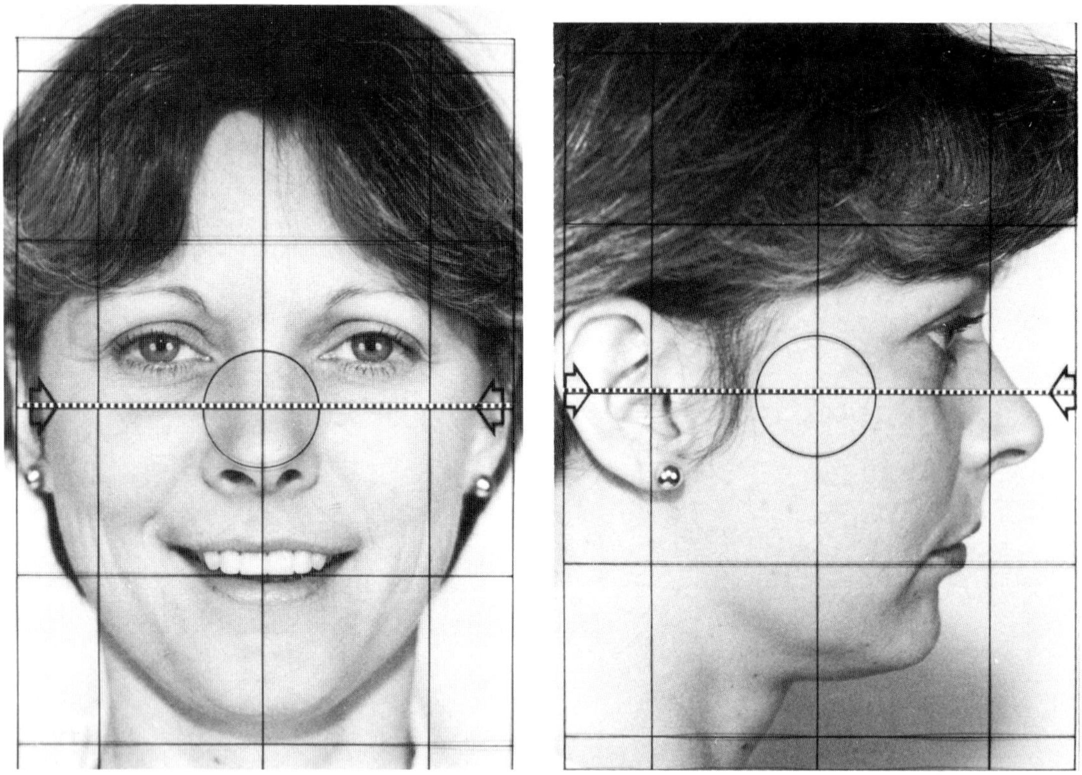

a b

Figure 5. **a,b,** The Frankfort horizontal line, traversing a horizontal plane through the top of the tragus and the infraorbital rim, is the single most important factor to consider when aligning the head for uniform positioning.

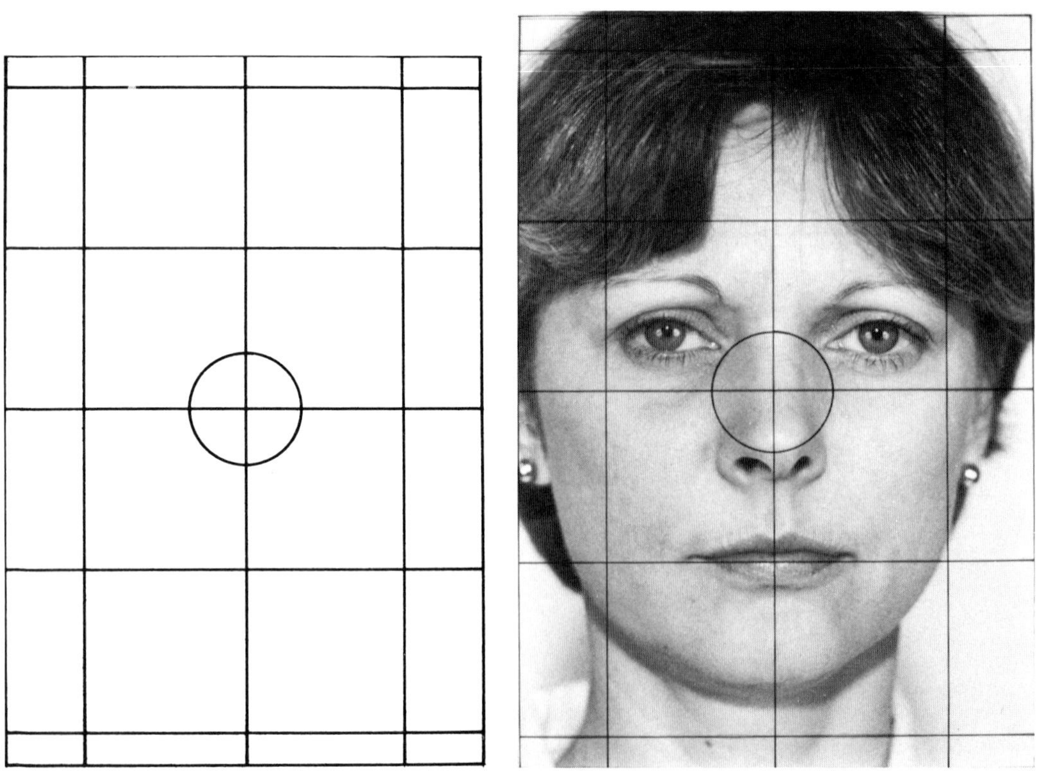

a b

Figure 6. **a,** Typical pattern of grid-viewing screen, invaluable in properly standardizing patient head alignment. **b,** Proper grid superimposition in frontal view, maintaining Frankfort horizontal line parallel to the floor. Midsagittal line is positioned in the midline to avoid head rotation. Equal amounts of the external ear should be visible.

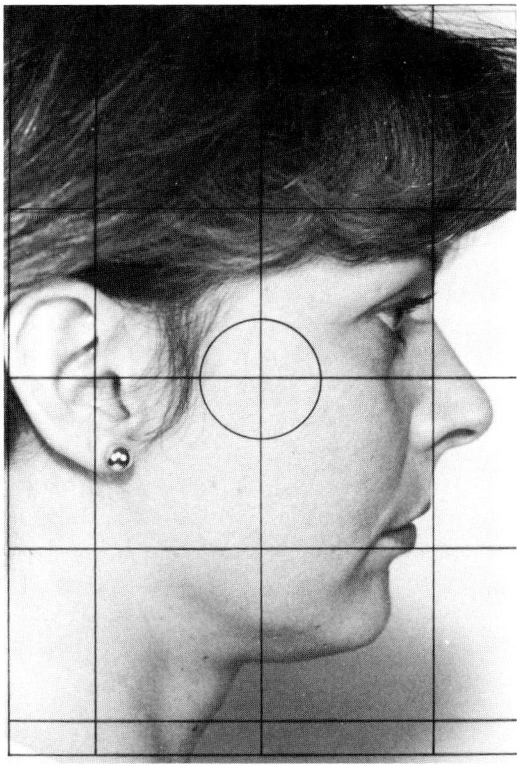

c

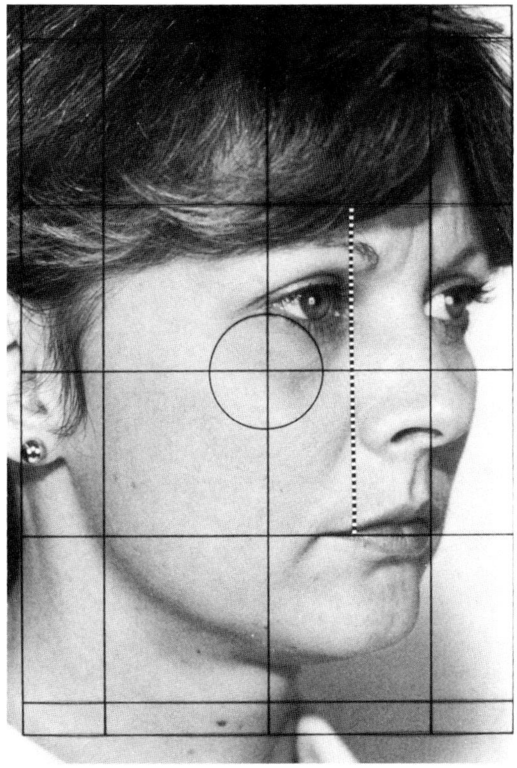

d

Figure 6. (*Continued*). **c,** Proper grid superimposition on lateral view. **d,** Proper grid superimposition on oblique view, with the vertical center grid lined up accurately with the inner canthus of the eye and the oral commissure. **e,** On base view, the nasal tip should ideally be positioned at a horizontal line passing through the interbrow area.

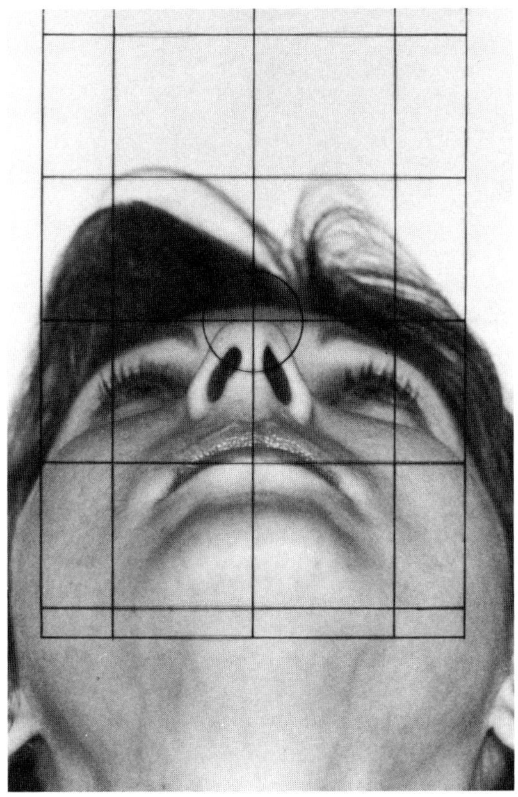

e

(submental) views are all facilitated by ensuring proper positioning of the head in relation to the Frankfort horizontal line.

Additional Framing Guidelines

Additional positioning factors must be appreciated when obtaining oblique and base views, involving positioning of the nasal tip. To ensure uniformity, the vertical center grid line should intersect and connect (or be aligned parallel to) the inner canthus with the oral commissure on oblique views (Fig. 6d), and for base views, the nasal tip should be positioned precisely at a horizontal line passing through the interbrow areas (Fig. 6e). Although the extent of tip projection may change slightly after rhinoplasty surgery, particularly when overprojected noses are repositioned or underprojected tips are augmented and rotated, in actual practice the difference is slight enough to create little appreciable variation in pre- and postoperative uniformity photograph positioning.

Many otherwise acceptable facial photographs are reduced in their value by failure to control the patient's hair (Fig. 7a). Hairstyles that obscure vital portions of the patient's facial anatomy often confuse the diagnostic and record-keeping process, reduce the quality of the image by absorbing large quantities of light (or, in the case of very fair individuals, reflecting too much light), obscure the desired background, and hide vital portions of the face.

Simple measures may be taken to reduce these possibilities. Hair clips, combs, elastic headbands and barrettes can be used during the photographic sitting to hold the hair away from the face temporarily (Fig. 7b-e). Colored elastic headbands are particularly effective in controlling the hair during photography for otoplasty (Fig. 8). Either method will allow the ear to be visualized during rhinoplasty and face-lift photography, allowing all vital features to be appreciated and the Frankfort horizontal line to be accurately sighted.

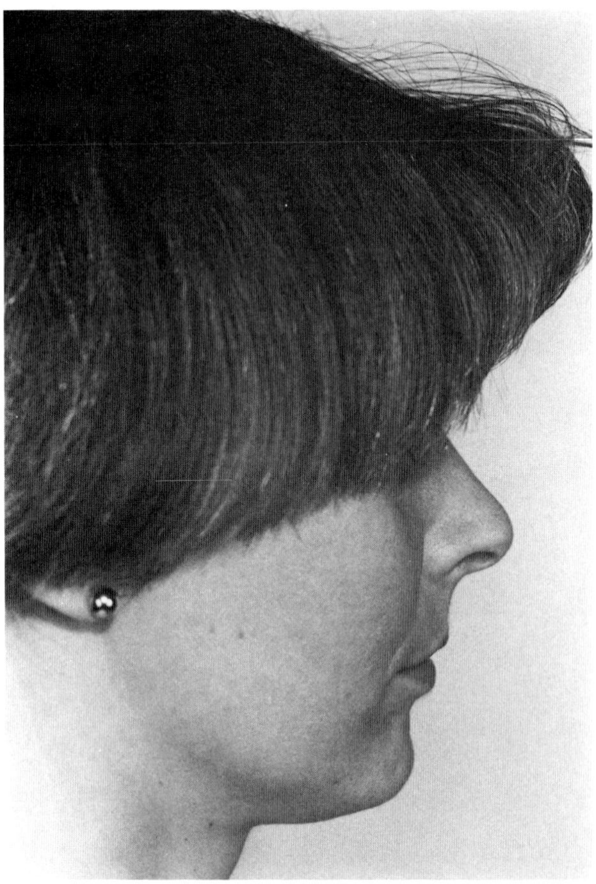

a

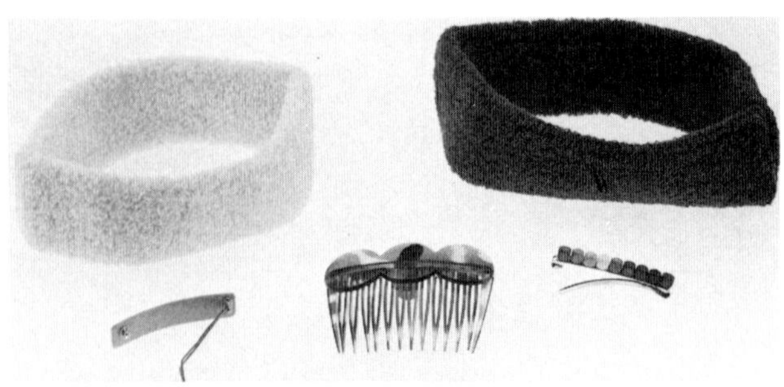

b

Figure 7. a, Uncontrolled hair in patient photographs is distracting and often obscures vital details of anatomy. **b–e,** Little effort is required to control the hair away from the face with the use of hair clips, pins, barrettes, combs, or headbands. Facial detail and proportion are now more clearly evident.

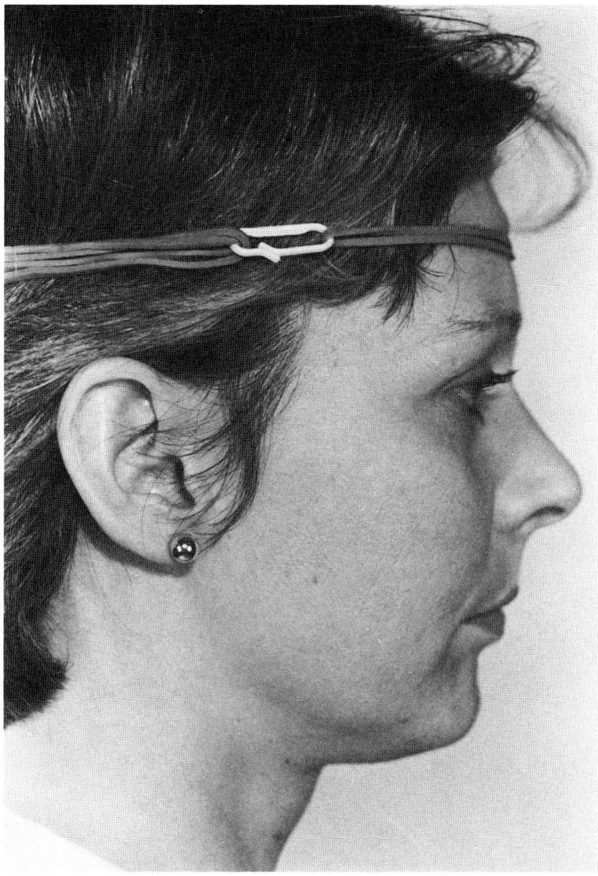
c

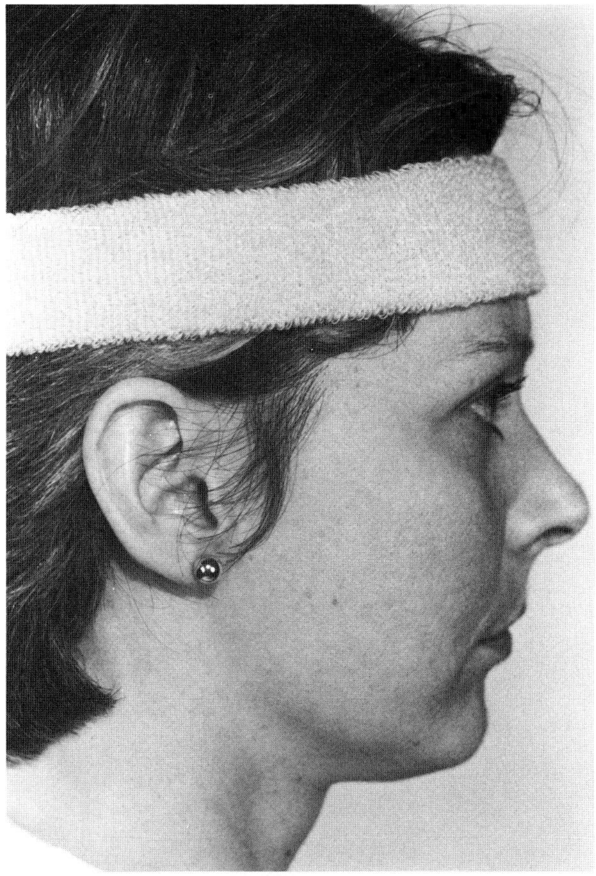
d

Figure 7. (*Continued*)

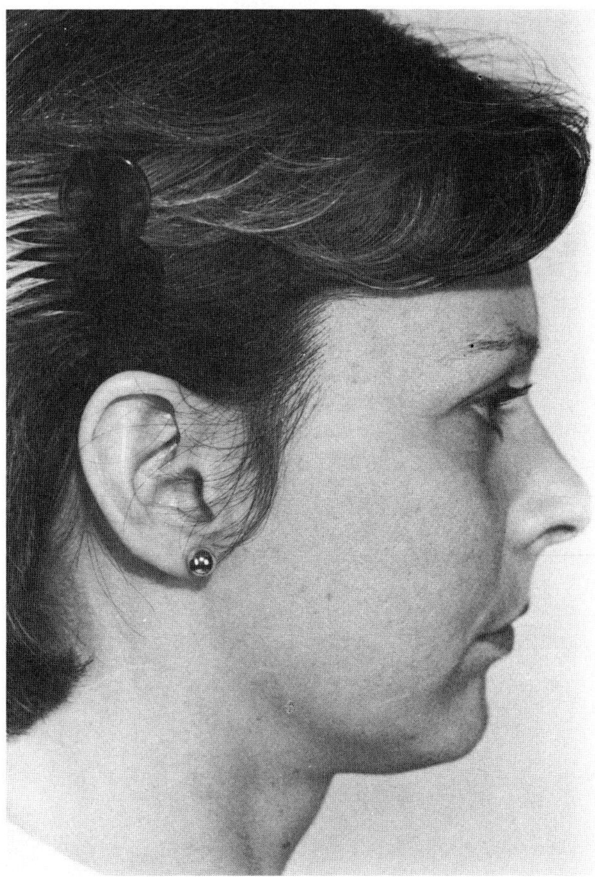
e

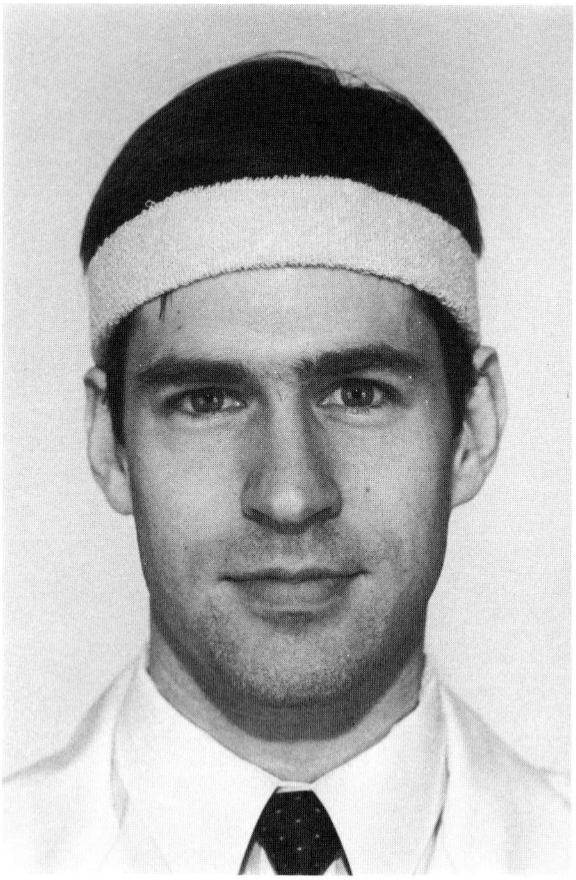
a

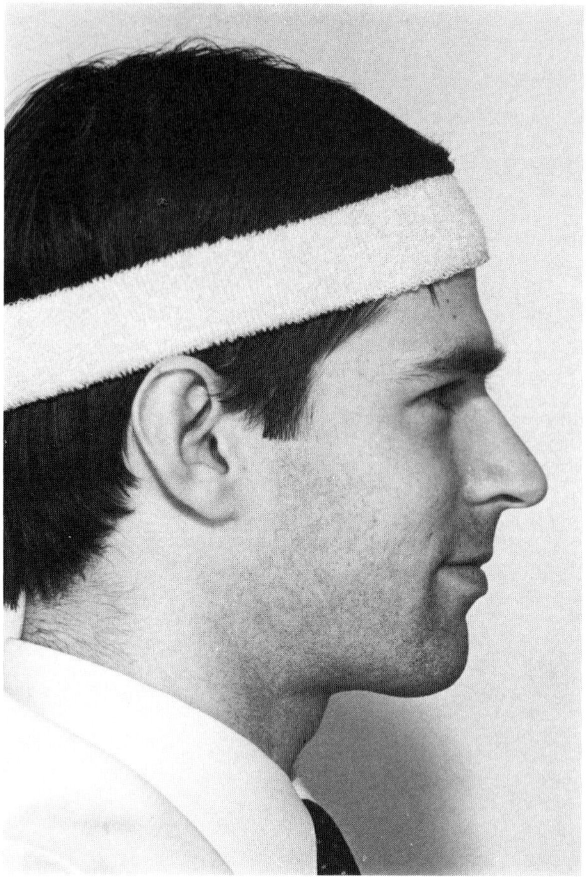
b

Figure 8. **a,b,** Particularly in patients undergoing otoplasty, controlling the hair with headbands is useful to gain full visualization of auricular position and attitude. The same elastic bands are quite useful as inconspicuous and colorful postoperative protective dressings.

Background

Many acceptable medical photographs are compromised by the appearance of a distracting, nonuniform background. This is unfortunate, since controlling the background is clearly one of the simplest tasks in medical photography. Improper backgrounds can distort the image, conceal vital information, disturb equal lighting, and distract from the main purpose of the photograph (Fig. 9).

In portrait photography, the most suitable background should be of a color complementary to skin tones. The photographer is not attempting to create special effects, but is striving to record patient information exactly as it appears to be, without embellishment or alteration of information.

In practice, light shades of blue or green seem to serve best for background (Fig. 10). The finish of the background should preferably be of a matte or dull appearance, partially absorbing and not reflecting light. It should be crease- and seam-free for perfect uniformity. No discernible pattern should be apparent to distract from the patient image.

As detailed in the section on lighting, it is ideal if the light reaching the background is augmented by a ceiling-mounted slave-triggered electronic flash (the "key" light or "kicker") to illuminate shadows and facilitate the impression of depth in the photograph (see Fig. 56). In addition, the top-mounted flash may slightly backlight the patient, further improving the illusion of depth and three dimensions.

White and gray are acceptable background colors, but they tend to be less complementary to skin tones than blue or green, and therefore they are less aesthetically pleasing. In addition, slides taken of patients with white or light gray backgrounds tend to reveal every particle of dust when projected.

Black and very dark backgrounds are poor choices in medical photography of patients (see Fig. 9a). Light is "swallowed up" to an unpleasant degree, the appearance of depth or third dimension is sacrificed, and the patient's image seems to be absorbed into the background. In profile views especially, the precise detail of the profile line is more difficult to distinguish. When converted into black

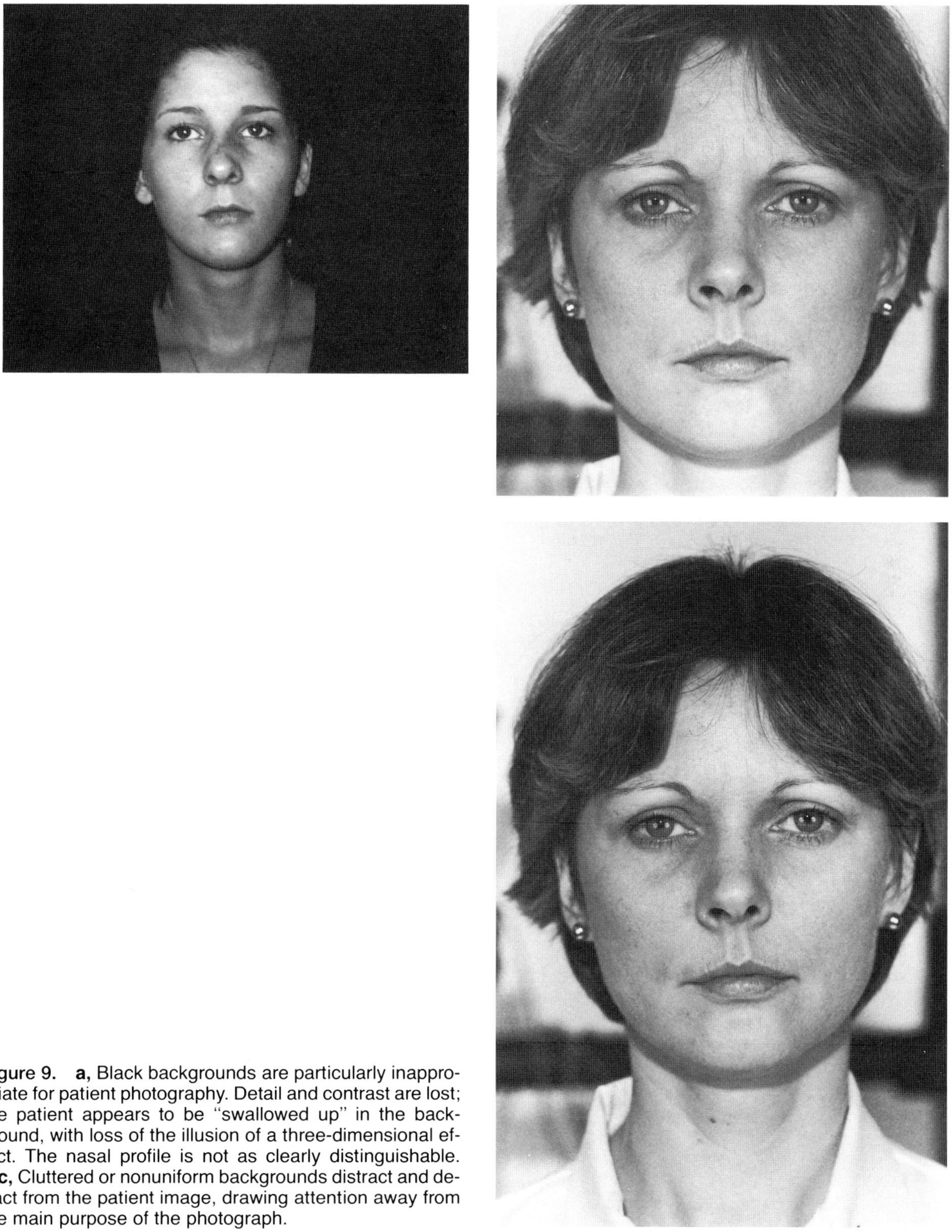

a

b

c

Figure 9. **a,** Black backgrounds are particularly inappropriate for patient photography. Detail and contrast are lost; the patient appears to be "swallowed up" in the background, with loss of the illusion of a three-dimensional effect. The nasal profile is not as clearly distinguishable. **b,c,** Cluttered or nonuniform backgrounds distract and detract from the patient image, drawing attention away from the main purpose of the photograph.

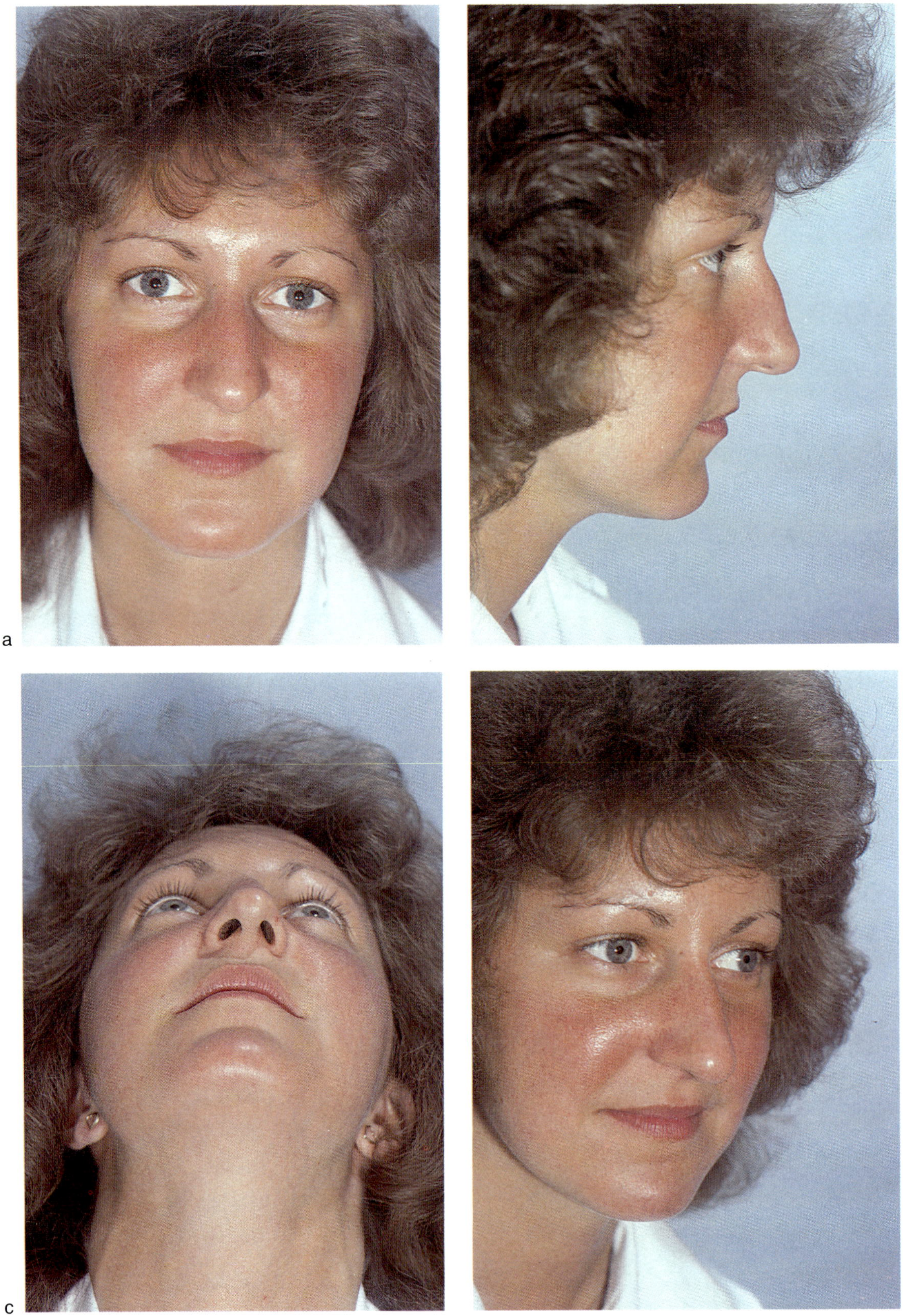

a b c d

Figure 10. a–d, Ideal backgrounds are complementary to skin tones, with light blue or green judged as best. They are nondistracting, uniform, and standard from sitting to sitting. They impart a lighter hue to the entire photograph while retaining good contrast and ensuring pleasing aesthetics.

and white prints for publication, photographs taken with black backgrounds are less distinct and contain less visual information than those with lighter backgrounds. For certain aspects of small-object photography, the black background is useful; in facial photography it should be abandoned.

A pleasing light blue background can be achieved in a variety of ways. In large photographic studios, seamless paper rolls of the desired color can be mounted above head height and unrolled to floor length. The paper is relatively inexpensive, and when soiled or in need of replacement, the mounted roll is simply unfurled further. In similar fashion, a suitably large section of this paper may be framed and mounted on the office wall as a stationary background. The background office wall itself may be painted the appropriate background shade, an inexpensive and practical alternative. Even simpler is the purchase of a simple plain-finish window shade of the proper size and color (Fig. 11), to be mounted on the wall as the photographic background.

Figure 11. Inexpensive window shades of appropriate complementary background colors can be purchased and mounted on a convenient office wall.

Controlling the background for medical photography, then, is simple; it is thus surprising how frequently in medical presentations and publications this fundamental principle is violated.

Proper creation and control of the background in the operating room is discussed in Chapter 3.

2 The Tools

CAMERA BODY

The introduction of the single-lens reflex (SLR) camera literally revolutionized the world of medical photography. Sophisticated 35 mm camera systems that possess capabilities for alternatives in photographic recording far beyond the needs for most medical photographers are available at very reasonable costs. Small, compact, lightweight, and durable camera bodies are produced by almost all major camera companies (Fig. 12); such a unit possesses obvious advantages in terms of weight, portability, durability, and ease of operation.

The important functions of the camera body in the overall photographic system include holding and transporting the film, providing an accurate viewing image of the subject, and, finally, recording the appropriate image when the shutter is released. SLR cameras offer the most extensive system of lenses and accessories, allowing flexibility plus professional quality results.

The image to be recorded by the SLR camera is transmitted through the camera lens onto an angled, movable mirror that transfers the image to a glass screen. No parallax error occurs, since the image is identical to the one received by the film. The image seen through the camera viewfinder by the photographer is therefore the image recorded, a distinct advantage in medical photography.

Our preference is for the Nikon system of cameras and lenses, and therefore the Nikon F series can be recommended (Fig. 13).

Durability and sturdiness are essential in any camera body used daily for literally thousands of exposures; in our experience Nikon products have endured well. Similar high-quality camera bodies from Canon, Olympus, Pentax, and others are available. The only defects experienced with camera bodies in the past decade have included breakage of the film advance lever mechanism (albeit after thousands of exposures; this problem can perhaps be minimized by use of a motor drive accessory) and "sticking" of the mirror mechanism (this can be minimized by avoiding exposure of the camera to dust and dirt and with occasional professional cleaning).

A critical feature of any camera is that it interface completely with the overall "system" of accessories chosen for medical photography.

CAMERA BODY ACCESSORIES

Accessories for photography are plentiful. Fundamentally, their use simply increases convenience and ease of operation, but none is indispensable for good medical photography. The surgeon-photographer just beginning practice may wish to add a certain number of these features as the volume of photography increases, for the sake of convenience, speed of operation, and, equally important, for personal pleasure.

"Soft Touch" Shutter Release Button

To prevent camera "shake" with consequent blurred images, a cable release (Fig. 14) is the ideal mechanism for tripping the shutter on cameras mounted on a tripod or stationary stand. A tripod-mounted camera, however, becomes inconvenient to use for a large volume and variety of medical photography, and therefore we prefer to hand-hold the camera to increase versatility of framing and angulation. Proper positions for hand-held cameras are well known and effective—we recommend their use (Fig. 15). The "soft touch" shutter release button constitutes a minimum investment which will further help to eliminate camera shake and preserve sharpness of detail.

For print copy work, slide duplication, and critical photography of small objects where versatility of camera position and speed of operation is less important, a stable camera tripod or mount with a cable release is, of course, preferred (Fig. 16).

Grid Focusing Screen

Most major 35 mm SLR cameras can be fitted with interchangeable focusing screens to accommodate special framing and focusing needs. Different forms

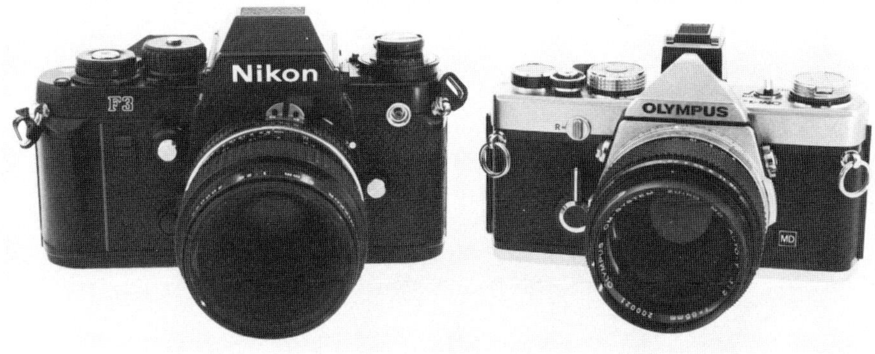

Figure 12. Compact, lightweight, and durable SLR cameras are produced by many major manufacturers. In developing a personal medical photography system, it is usually prudent to acquire component parts (camera body, lenses, etc.) made by the same manufacturer to ensure easy compatibility.

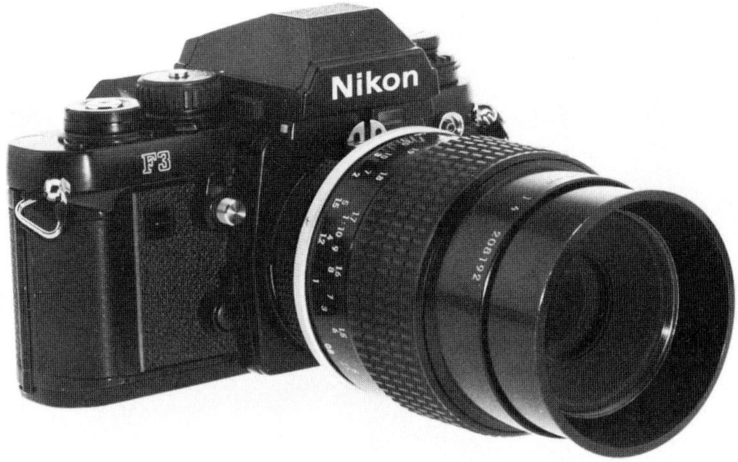

Figure 13. The Nikon system is unexcelled for sophistication and ease of use in medical photography.

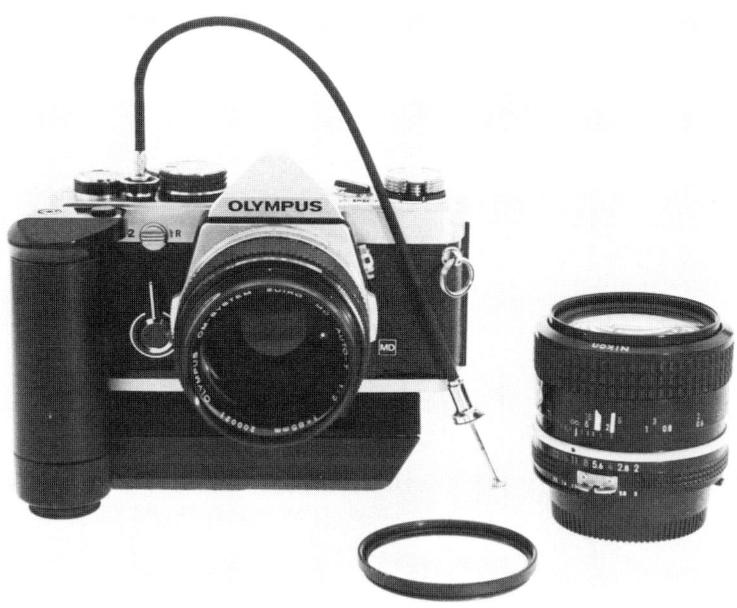

Figure 14. Cable release mounted on the camera body is used to eliminate camera shake.

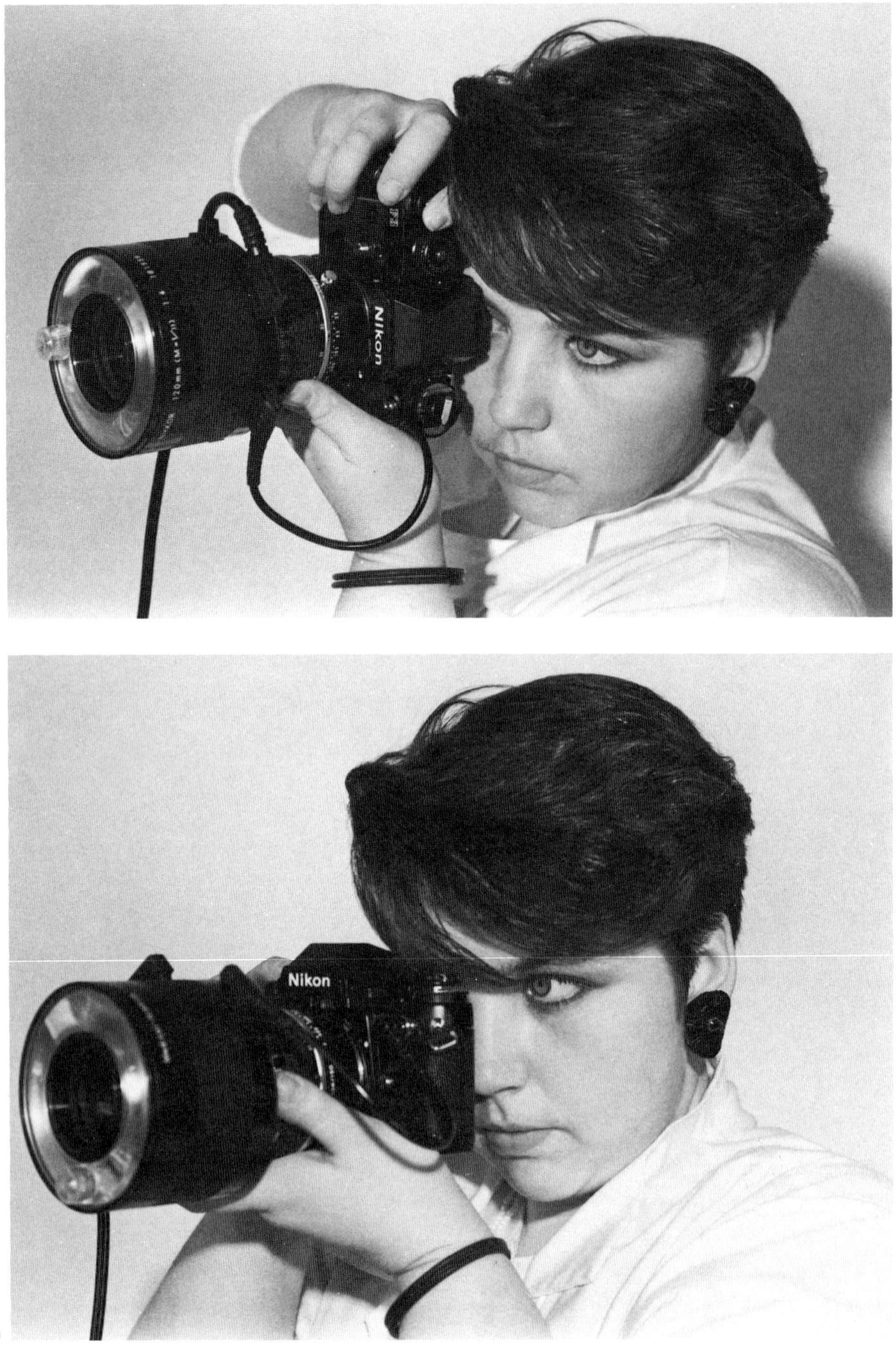

a

b

Figure 15. a,b, Various techniques for ensuring stability during hand-held photography. All incorporate a stable position of both hands relative to the camera. Locking one or both elbows into the body before releasing the shutter aids in camera stability.

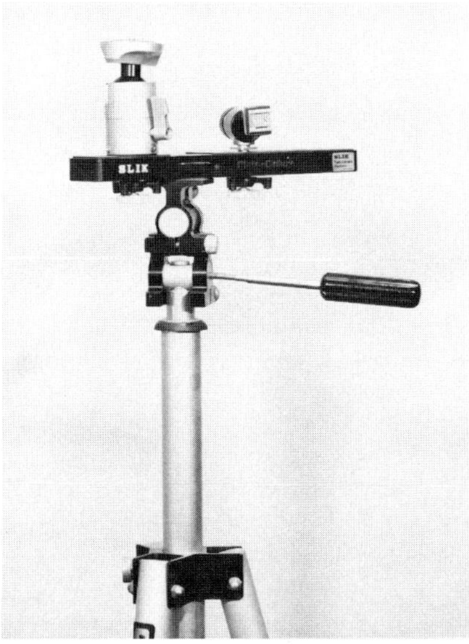

Figure 16. The camera tripod may be beneficial in critical photography of small objects and still images; in patient office photography we prefer to hand-hold the camera for flexibility and economy of time.

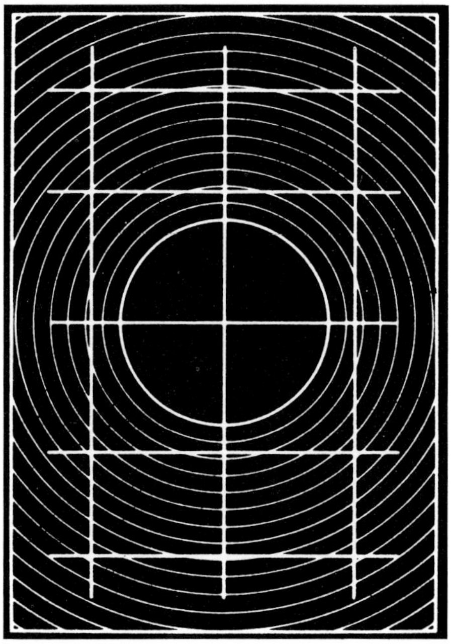

Figure 17. The typical configuration of the grid viewing screen.

of split-image screens are common; we prefer the gridded focusing screen (Fig. 17) to aid in proper facial positioning and alignment for standardization and uniformity, the ultimate goal of all medical photography. The grid pattern is used to ensure that the Frankfort horizontal line is observed (Fig. 18) and that the patient's face and head are truly vertical, avoiding tilting or angulation to one side (Fig. 19).

Motor Drive

Automatic film winders and motor drives (battery operated) are a convenience and not a necessity for accurate medical photography (Fig. 20). Motor drives are most efficient when employed for the rapid, undelayed recording of photographs in the surgical suite (Fig. 21), where time becomes more important. Multiple exposures can be made rapidly at different aperture settings ("bracketing") without removing the photographer's eye from the viewfinder or pausing to advance the film manually. Care must be taken, however, to avoid shooting too quickly before the electronic flash unit has completely recycled; otherwise, underexposed photographs will result (it is always prudent to allow 2 additional seconds after the onset of the ready light glow before tripping the shutter).

In addition, motor drives seem to save wear and tear on the film advance lever, a source of potential eventual breakdown in even the best equipment. The surgeon-photographer must simply weigh the cost-benefit-convenience factors of the motor drive in his work against the added expense and inconvenience of battery replacement to power the unit. In general, automatic winders are less expensive, whereas motor drives, due to their faster operating rates, are more versatile but also more costly.

Data-Back

The standard camera back may be replaced or augmented easily with a device called a data-back (Fig. 22); selected data are imprinted onto the film each time a frame is exposed (Fig. 23). The date, time, shutter speed, aperture, and other more personal codes, preselected by the photographer, can be imprinted. Dates of pre- and postoperative pictures are particularly useful if the surgeon is involved in a large amount of teaching. Precise data imprinted on the photograph can be a convenience for storage and retrieval systems, particularly those amenable to microcomputer information storage. Data-backs add significantly to the overall weight of the system and slightly to the bulkiness. Each data-back is ordinarily system-specific; each company produces a data-back compatible only with its own equipment system.

Carrying Case

If valuable cameras and lenses are moved frequently (for example, from an office to a hospital

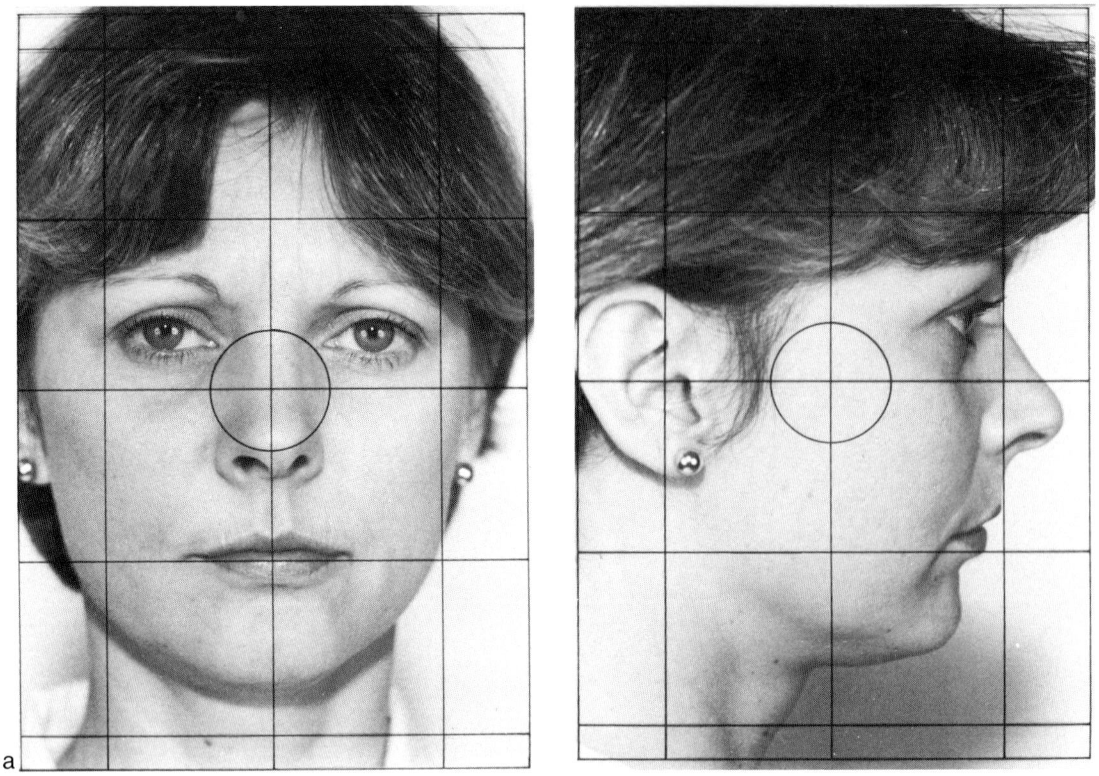

a b

Figure 18. a,b, Grid viewing screen is invaluable in accurately aligning the Frankfort horizontal line with the appropriate patient landmarks.

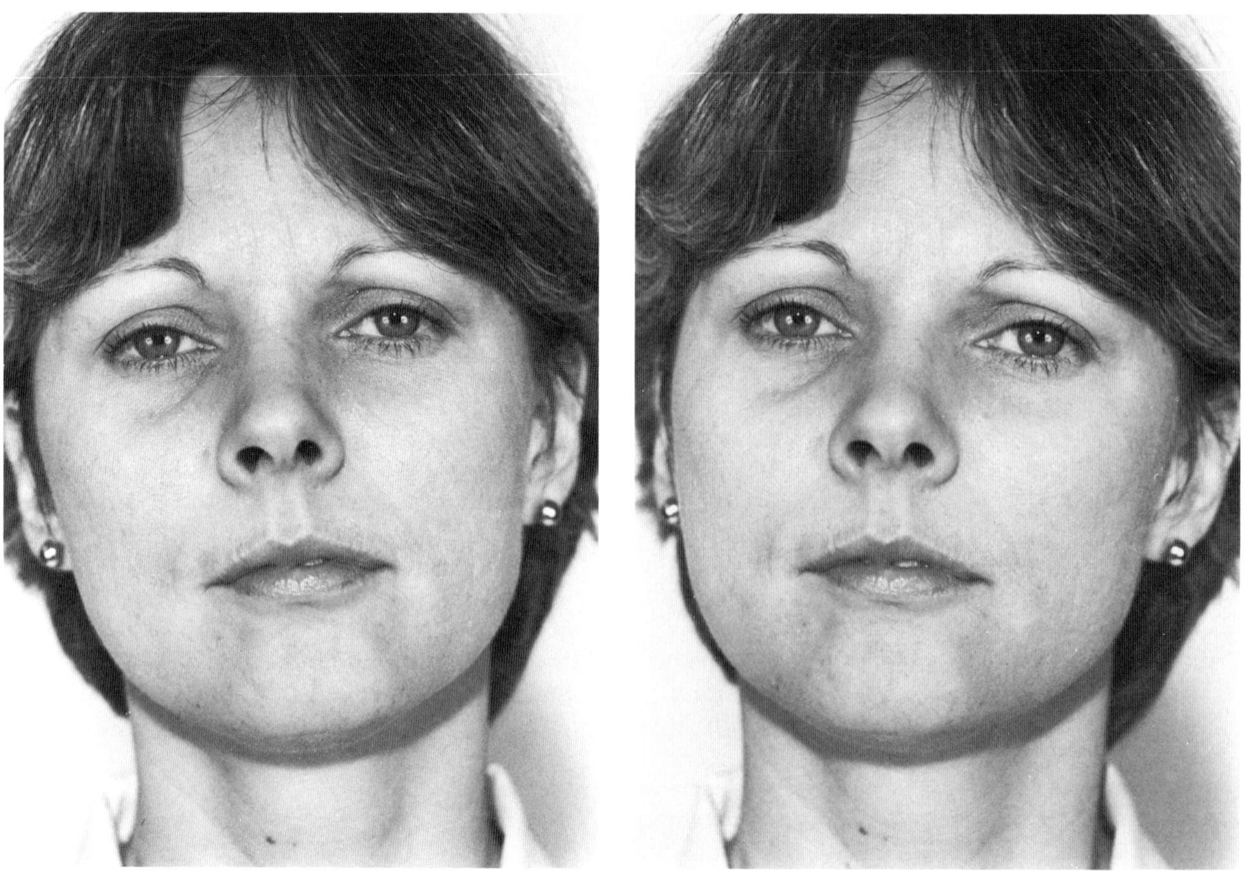

a b

Figure 19. a,b, Tilted and aberrant head positions common in nonstandardized patient photography.

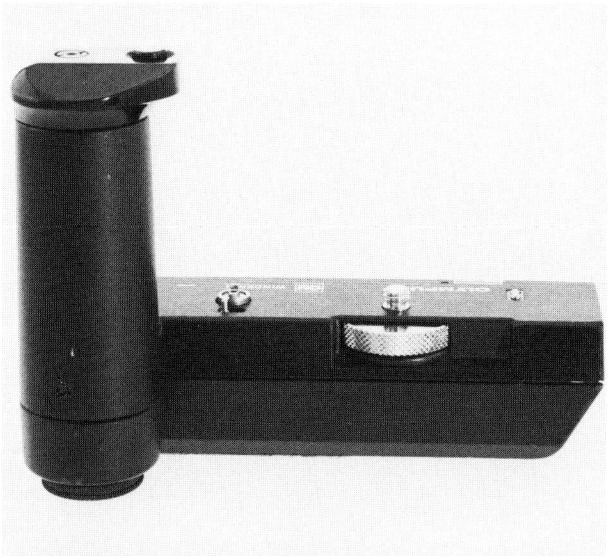

Figure 20. Typical motor drive unit designed to interface on base of camera body.

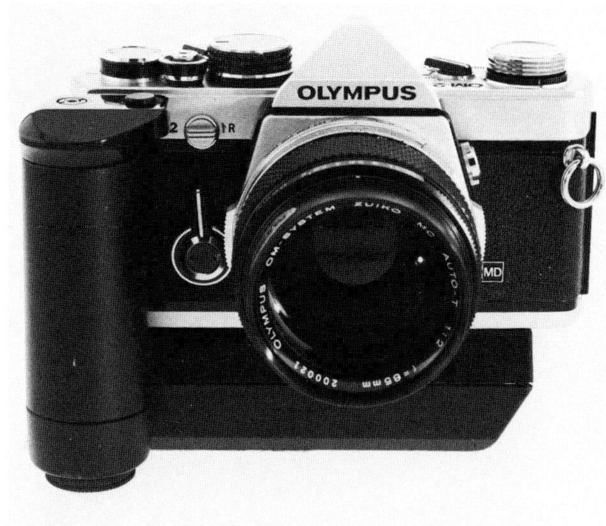

Figure 21. Motor drive interfaced to camera body.

operating room), it is wise to select a suitable carrying case for convenience and safety.

The hard-cover, foam rubber lined metal case made by Haliburton and others is ideal (Fig. 24). It is durable, highly protective, and serves to shield against moisture. Although somewhat more expensive than other cases, it will endure for many years with proper care. (Because it looks like a camera case, however, it may be more susceptible to theft than other less easily identifiable cases.) The lack of a shoulder strap may reduce its appeal slightly.

A suitable, less expensive alternative, also lightweight and durable, is the light nylon backpack custom fitted with foam rubber cushioning (Fig. 25). This unit can be custom designed by its user to fit specific needs to house individual pieces of equipment. A waterproof pack is best, form fitted with high-quality foam rubber. Cutouts in the foam rubber are most easily and most accurately created with a standard kitchen electric knife (Fig. 26). Such "homemade" cases withstand even severe vibration and trauma and are ideal for outdoor pho-

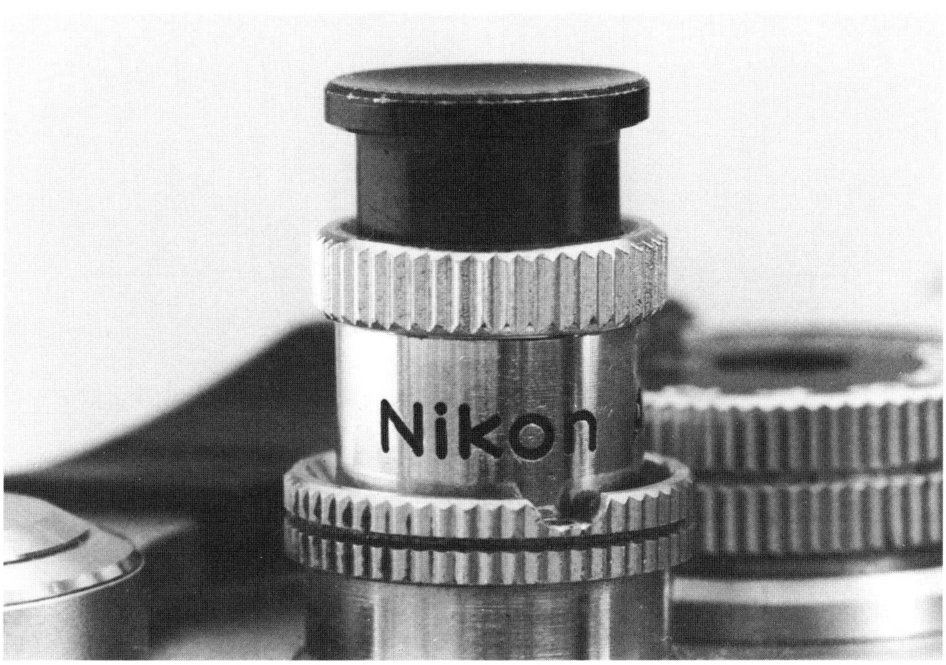

Figure 22. Typical data-back unit.

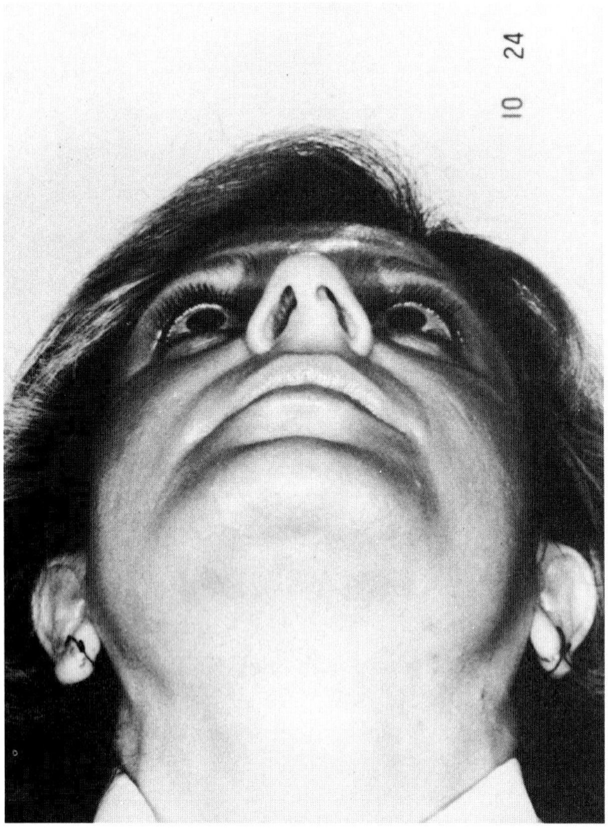

Figure 23. Imprinted data on 2 × 2 slide can be useful in teaching as well as in efficient cataloguing and storage of slides.

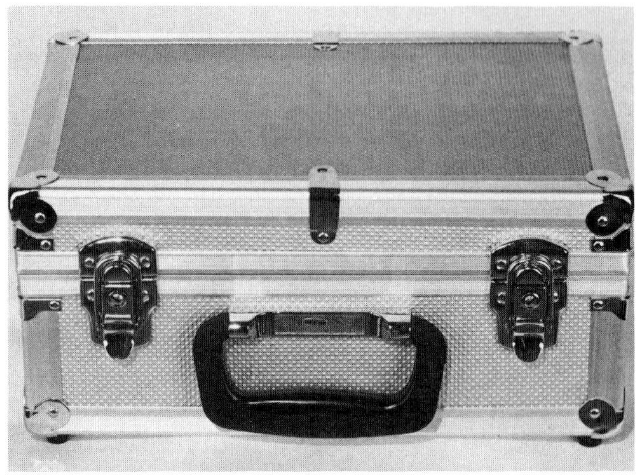

Figure 24. Lightweight, sturdy metal camera case.

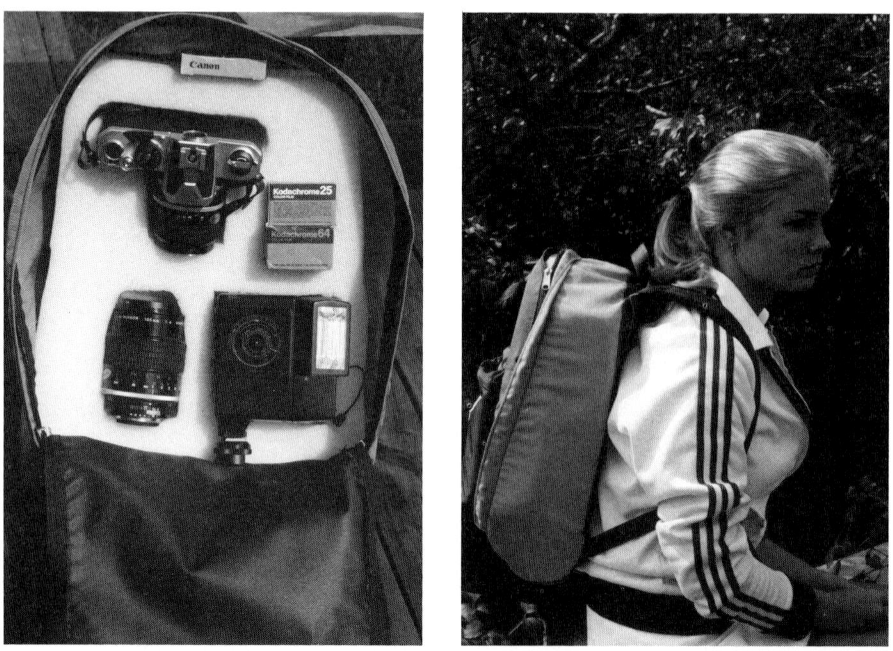

a b

Figure 25. **a,b,** Light nylon backpack cushioned with custom-contoured foam rubber.

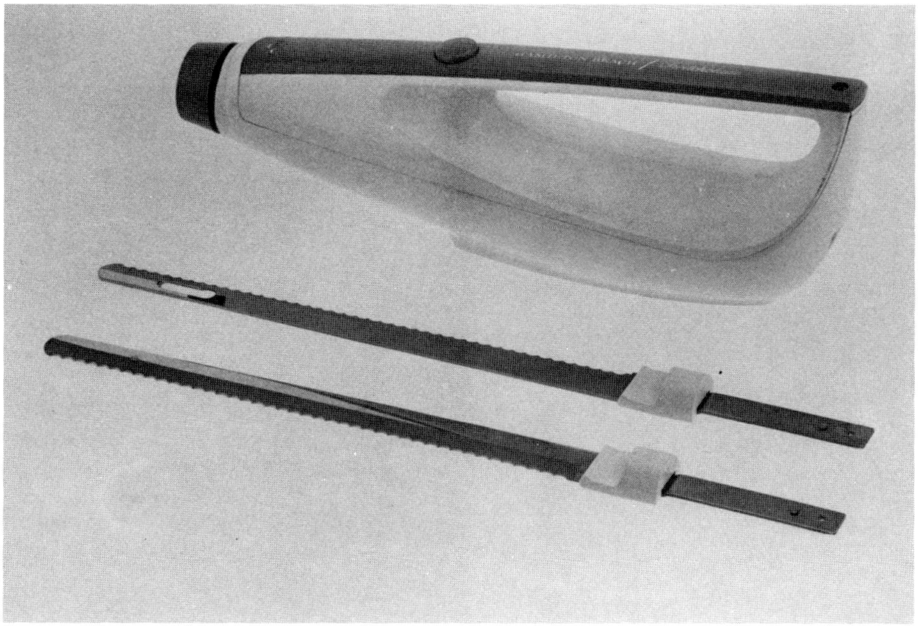

a

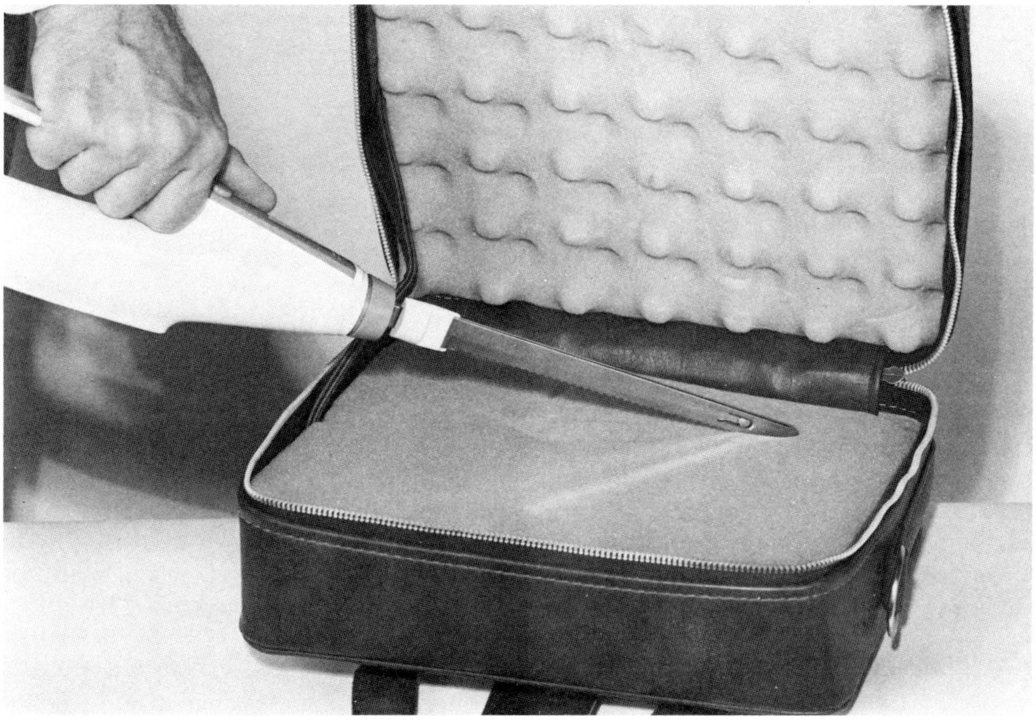

b

Figure 26. a,b, The oscillating kitchen knife is the most precise instrument for custom contouring the foam cushion in camera cases. Faultless cutouts can be individually created for each piece of camera equipment.

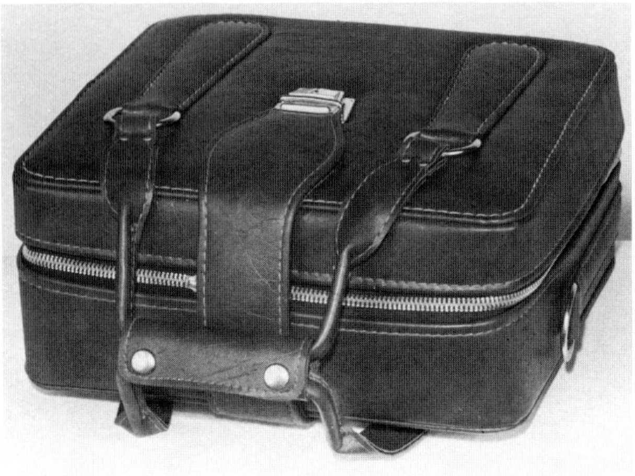

Figure 27. Soft camera case with shoulder strap.

tographic adventures. In addition, the ubiquitous backpack attracts less attention than more traditional camera cases, providing further protection against theft.

For protecting a single camera and lens, the standard army ammunition case, form fitted internally with foam rubber, also provides extreme protection from damage and moisture for the outdoor photographer or for the photographer transporting camera equipment in the trunk of a car.

Soft gadget bags of all varieties and descriptions exist (Fig. 27). Their light weight and shoulder strap render them easily portable, but some designs tend toward equipment disorganization.

Photographic consent forms should be stored in the camera case for use in emergency room situations (or in any other setting in which prior consent to photography may not have been obtained (Fig. 28). Clear, informed consent for photography must be obtained, and witnessed, from every patient or responsible guardian before receiving any medication. Failure to follow this all-important principle may lead to the eruption of an unwanted and unnecessary lawsuit.

In the final analysis, the surgeon-photographer should survey what is available and select a protective case that best suits individual needs, budget, and photographic plans. Camera protection is a wise investment.

LENSES

The quality and characteristics of the lens used in medical photography is perhaps the most critical link in the photographic system. Whereas some "corner cutting" may be acceptable (or photographically imperceptible) in the selection of other basic elements of the system, no compromise

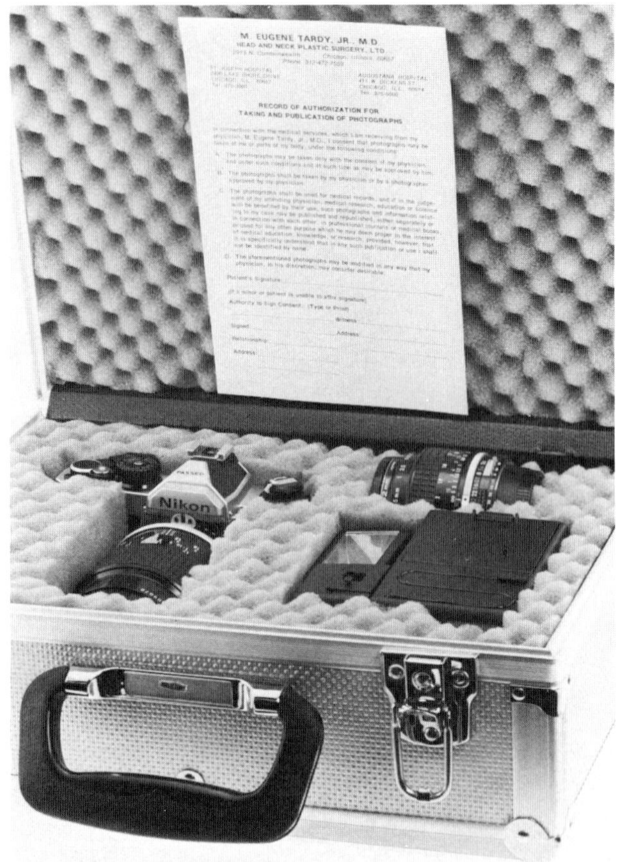

Figure 28. Storing photographic consent forms in the lid of the camera carrying case is particularly convenient, particularly when photographs are required in an emergency situation.

should be allowed in selection of the best possible lens.

The standard lens in the typical 35 mm system is usually about 50 mm. If used for patient photography, it creates unpleasant and inaccurate parallax distortion in facial portraits (Fig. 29) and thus significantly limits its use. Ideally, the "medium" telephoto lenses, particularly those designated "macro" and possessing longer focal lengths, serve best for accurate photographic recording. Medium telephoto lenses (90 to 105 mm) are ideally suited for portrait photography because they minimize facial distortion and allow a comfortable working distance between the patient and photographer while providing a full-frame image (Fig. 30).

In a medical office, where space for a photographic set-up is usually limited, the 105 mm Auto Micro-Nikkor telephoto lens is an ideal choice (Fig. 31). Relatively fast lenses (F/2 or F/2.8) are available, and, again, no compromise should be made in the selection of the best lens compatible with the overall system. For the majority of facial photography, the 105 mm lens may be racked out to its

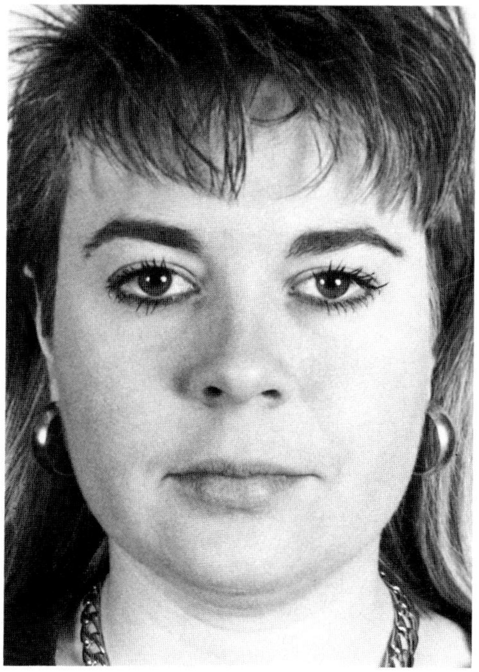

Figure 29. Head shots taken with the standard 50 mm lens creates sufficient parallax distortion of the facial image to be inaccurate and displeasing.

maximum focal length for complete standardization and uniformity of distance and image size. From sitting to sitting, then, all patient photographs will be of exactly the same dimensions (Fig. 32).

For close-up views (scars, lesions, orbit), predetermined distances may be marked on the lens to ensure distance uniformity for each of these specific views (Fig. 33).

The 105 mm macro lens is ideal for surgical photography, since the medium telephoto length allows close-up views without compromise of sterility in the surgical suite. The photographer can remain a comfortable distance from the field of interest and yet document close-ups with relative ease (Fig. 34).

For more extreme close-up photography (skin lesion, scars, implants, foreign bodies, and other small objects) the 55 mm macro lens can be useful (Fig. 35). In addition, it functions well for flat copy work from books, illustrations, and photographs (Fig. 36).

All lenses should be protected from dirt, smudges, and abrasions by mounting a clear ultraviolet or skylight filter over the exposed lens (Fig. 37A,B). This small investment can be very important, considering the expense of good fast lenses.

a

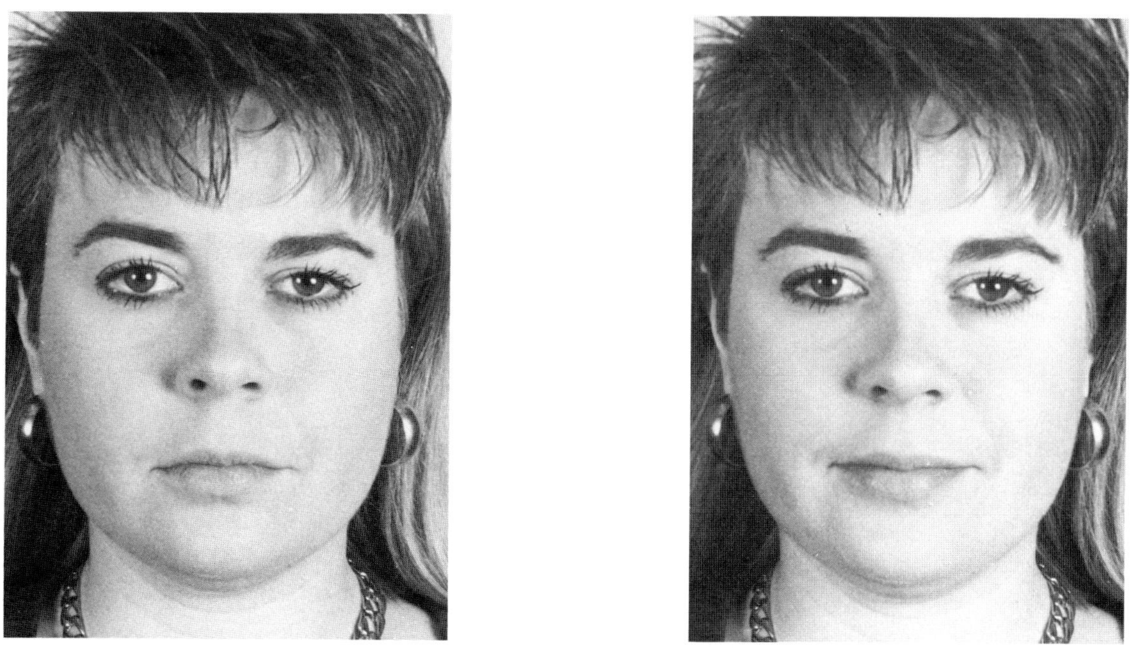

b

Figure 30. **a,** Head shots taken with the 90 mm lens overcomes the problem of parallax distortion, but the image obtained is not as accurate as desired. **b,** The ideal head or face image is obtained with the 100 mm or 105 mm lens, accurately reproducing facial proportions and providing sharpness without distortion.

Before purchasing any lens, the buyer should be absolutely sure that it is mount-compatible with the camera system for which it is to be used.

FILM

Among the myriad types of film available for photography, the Kodachromes set the standard for the industry today (Fig. 38). Both Kodachrome 25 and 64 produce color transparencies of faithful color, extremely fine grain (and therefore sharp images), and stable emulsions, all absolute prerequisites for ultimate quality in medical photography. These laudable characteristics translate into significant advantages for the facial surgeon. If enlargements of the transparency are to be made (for publication or exhibits), the fine grain of the Kodachromes allows significant enlargement without noticeable loss of sharp detail. Color slides lend themselves better than any other format to storage, retrieval, and cataloguing, a significant advantage when a slide library numbers in the thousands or tens of thousands. In medical education, the 2 × 2 slide transparency represents the current world standard, and slide projectors (ordinarily the carousel slide projector or its close equivalent) are found in almost every teaching institution in the world.

Perhaps more faithfully than any photographic film available, the Kodachromes reproduce colors representative of human skin tones. Batches of film developed in Kodak emulsion processing possess the longest archival retention of true colors than any other film by far (testing laboratories have assigned an estimate of at least a 50-year stability for Kodachrome emulsions when stored under proper conditions of relative darkness, low humidity, and stable cool temperatures). This is substantiated by our experience, since K-25 slides taken 20 years ago and projected scores of times in relatively hot projectors still retain true and faithful colors.

Finally, color slides are the most economical of all photographs, thus encouraging the photographer to be generous in the number of exposures he makes in important shooting situations. Since slides are easily and accurately reproduced (and even enhanced) rapidly and faithfully in modern slide reproduction units (the ChromoPro and the Illumitron units serve admirably for this purpose) (Fig. 39), copies can be quickly made for teaching and publishing purposes, while the original may be properly stored under stable conditions for archival purposes.

A further major advantage of the slide transparency is its use for ready reference in the operating room. Projecting in life size and in full color the patient's photographs in the operating room during surgery provides the ultimate in moment-to-

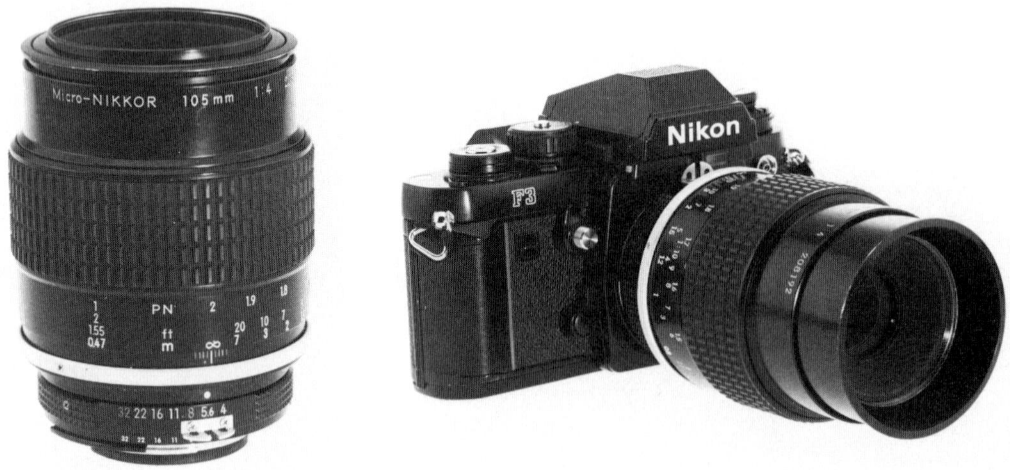

a b

Figure 31. **a,b,** The 105 mm Auto Micro-Nikkor lens is ideal for both patient portrait photography as well as close-up and operating room photography.

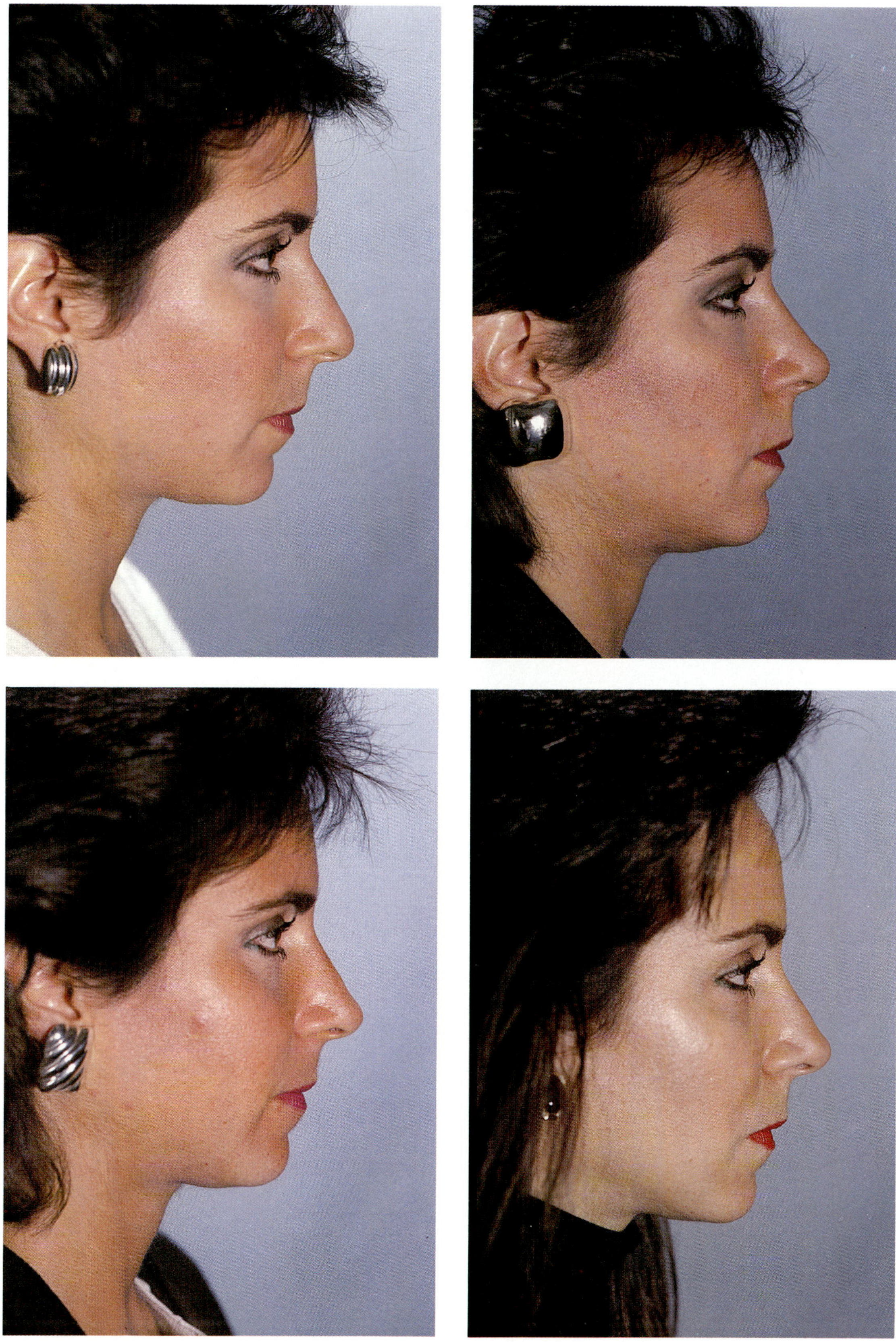

a b c d

Figure 32. Uniform patient photographs from sitting to sitting result from the use of the 105 mm lens, as in this patient recorded (a) preoperative, (b) at 1 week, (c) at 6 months, and (d) at 12 months.

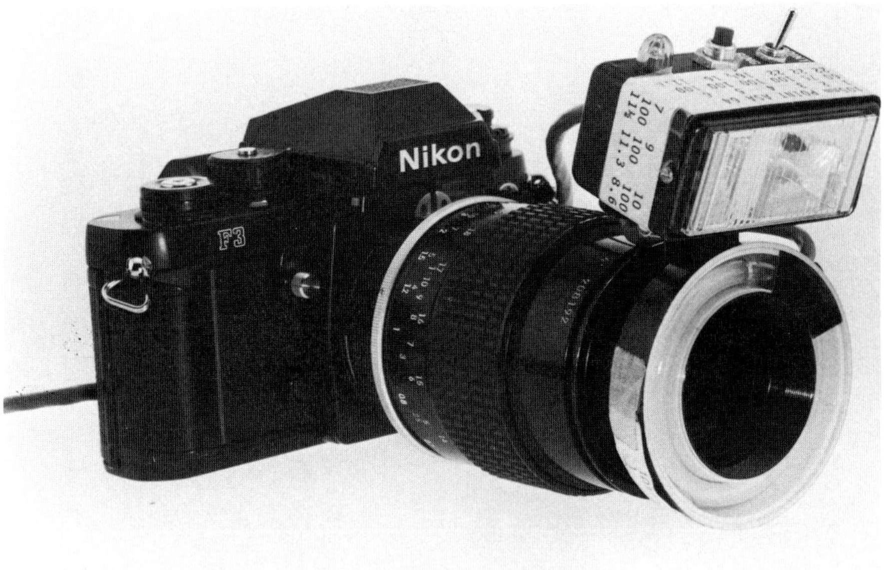

a

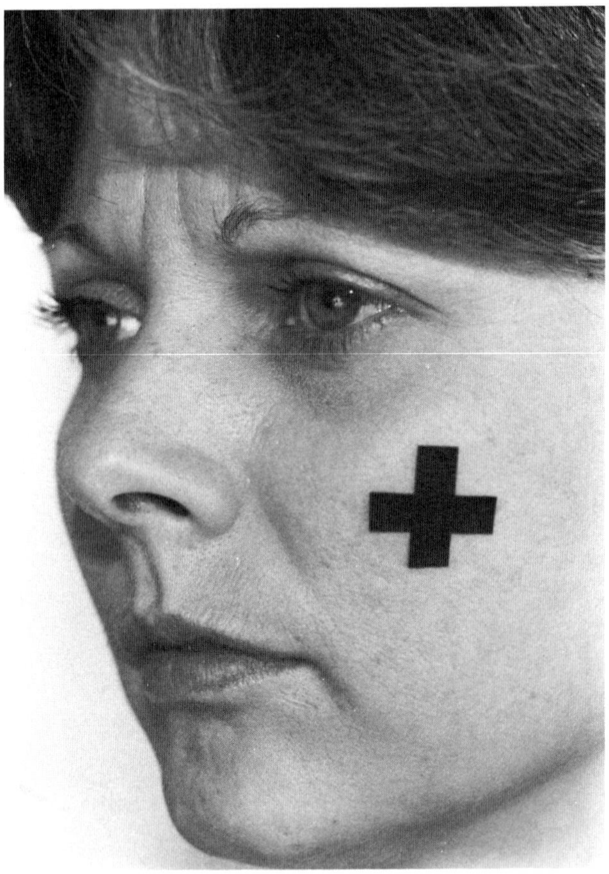

b

Figure 33. **a,** Predetermined distance markings placed on the lens help to supplement the manufacturer's codings, thus reminding the photographer from shot to shot of proper distances for standardization and uniformity. **b,** Close-up view taken with the 105 mm lens.

moment comparisons of minute and critical details during the surgical procedure (Fig. 40). Very little extra effort and equipment is required to achieve this added refinement to careful surgery, whereas improved teaching during the operative procedure is a major benefit to the observer.

One significant drawback to the regular use of the Kodachromes does exist. Development for the most part must be carried out in Kodak processing laboratories. Although this requirement ensures a reliable degree of quality control, it is time-consuming and frustrating to the surgeon requiring the results of his exposed photographic rolls as quickly as possible.

Shooting Kodak Ektachrome film allows the development of a usable slide within just a few hours, which may be a major advantage when color transparencies are urgently needed and long-term reten-

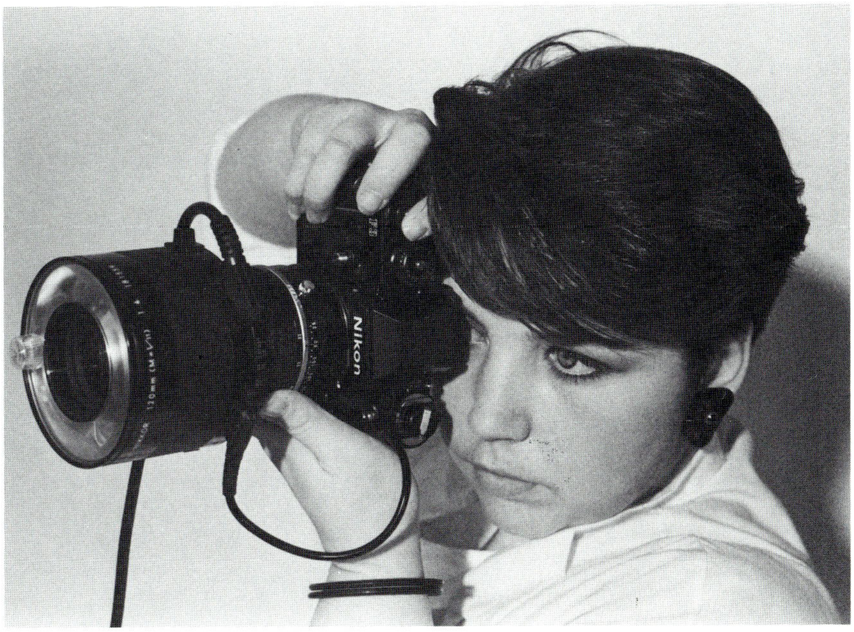

Figure 34. In the operating room, use of the 105 mm lens provides a comfortable working distance from the sterile operating field for long as well as close shots.

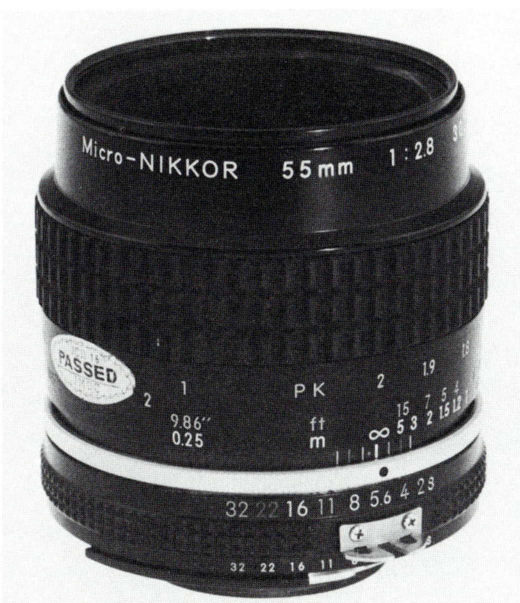

Figure 35. A useful alternative for medical close-up work is the Auto Micro-Nikkor 55 mm lens, useful for small skin lesions, scars, extreme detail, and for print copy work.

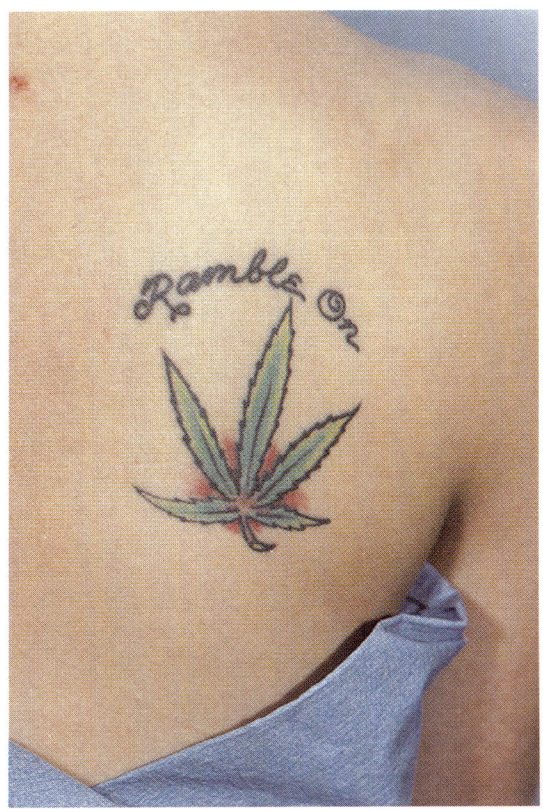

Figure 36. Close-up photograph recorded with the 55 mm Auto Micro-Nikkor lens.

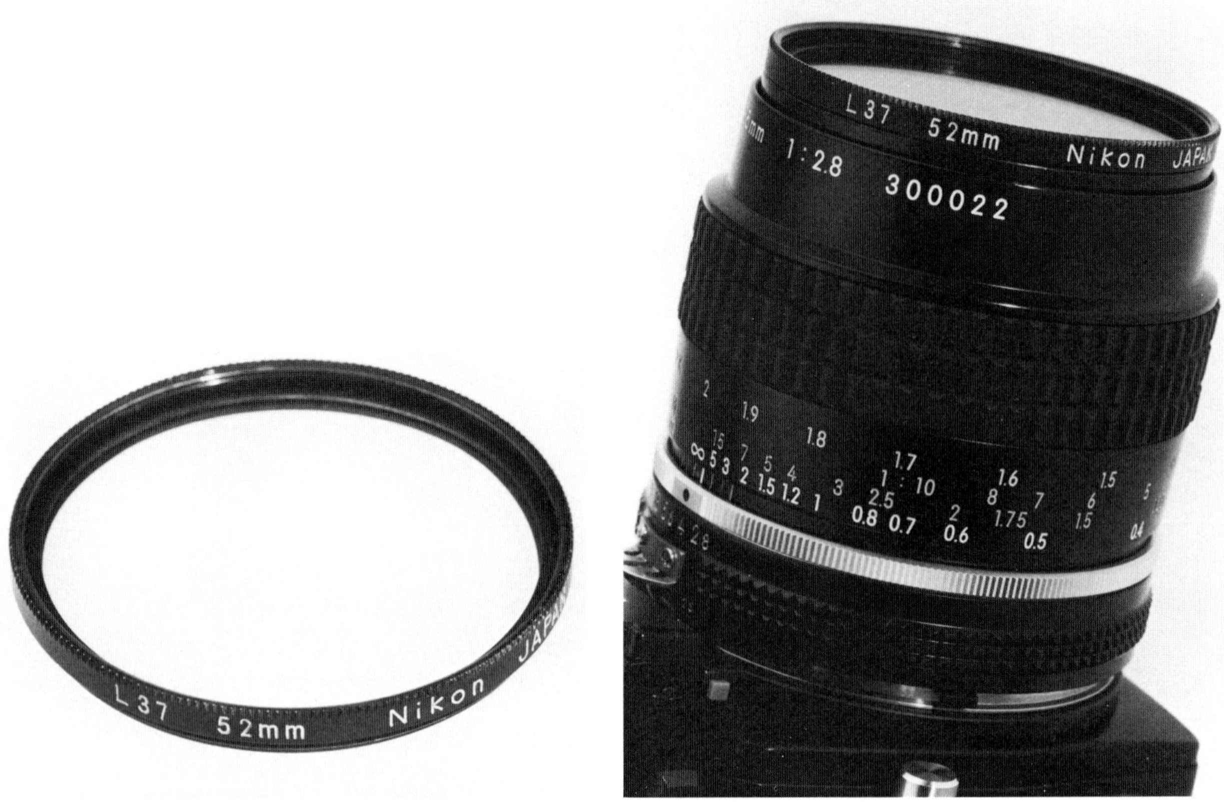

a b

Figure 37. a,b, All expensive lenses should be protected by mounting a clear ultraviolet or skylight filter to the lens. The filter thus protects the lens from dust, and it can be inexpensively replaced if damaged.

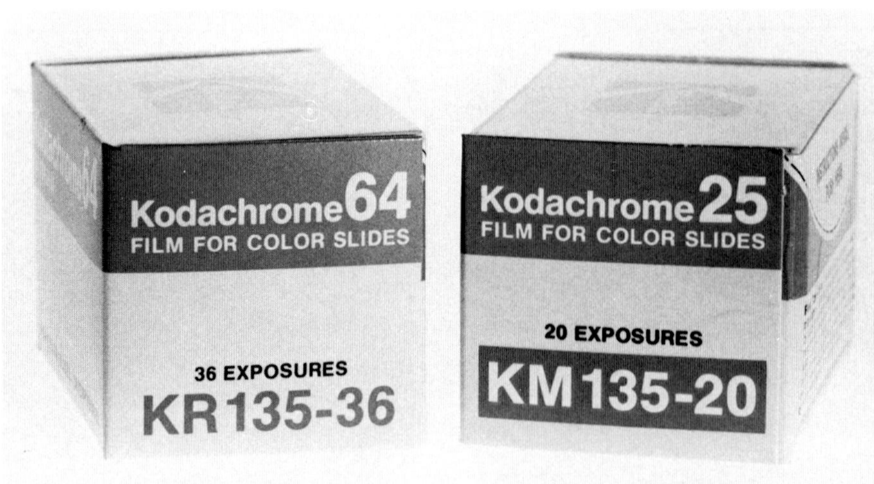

Figure 38. The Kodachromes represent the standard by which all other films for routine medical use are judged. In an office or operating room situation, they are universally the films of choice.

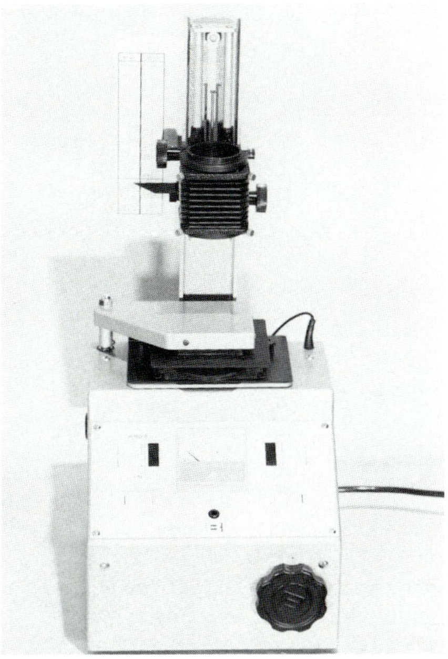

Figure 39. Modern slide copy units are marvels of engineering, allowing very accurate and faithful slide reproduction along with the creation of many different and unique slide combinations for teaching or publication.

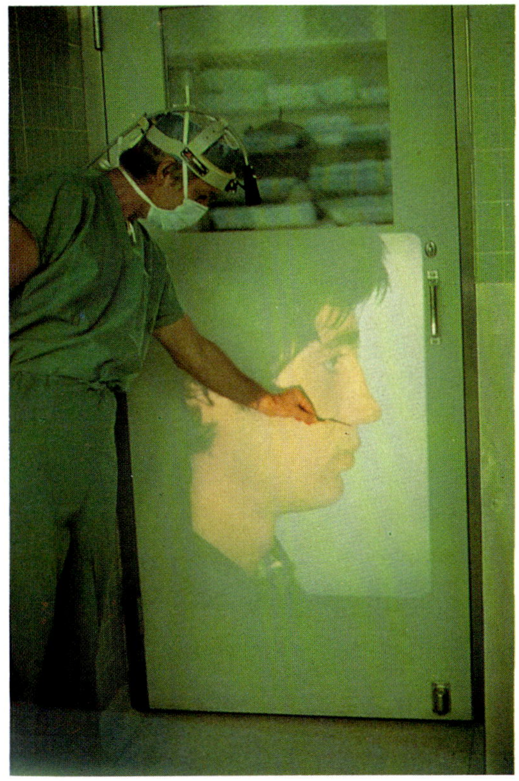

Figure 40. Color slides of patients projected in greater than life size in the operating room during surgery allow the most accurate and critical comparison available, aesthetically, to the surgeon. Intraoperative teaching is facilitated, since overlays of white paper can be temporarily superimposed over the projected image and proposed procedures and techniques discussed.

tion of stable colors and hues is not as critical (Ektachrome dyes deteriorate much more quickly than Kodachrome, and fade significantly when projected frequently or exposed to ordinary light for a relatively short period of time). For this reason, we use Ektachrome slides only when transparencies are required within a matter of hours and long-term storage and archival retention is unimportant.

An adjunctive system, providing a back-up capability and an instant printed image, is the Polaroid system of cameras and film (Fig. 41). It can be quite useful to record two or more instant Polaroid shots during the initial patient consultation (a frontal and lateral view usually will suffice). These photographs are not of the quality and sharpness inherent in the slide transparency, but they can be a valuable visual springboard to facilitate communication between the patient and the surgeon. In addition, they can be filed in the patient's chart for ready evaluation at subsequent visits (Fig. 42) and ultimately may be presented to the patient sometime in the postoperative period, a courtesy ordinarily greatly appreciated. Polaroid prints by themselves are only an adjunct to the more refined photographs described, and they are not acceptable as the only system of photographic recording to be used. In addition, they are expensive.

Relatively instant color Polaroid prints may be produced from 2 × 2 slides obtained with the recommended standardized system. Slide-to-print copy units manufactured by Polaroid (the Polaprinter) and Vivitar are inexpensive and simple to use (Fig. 43). Such prints are useful for filing and patient review, as well as for insurance and legal records.

Other more specialized films are useful in the wide range of medical photography. These special applications are discussed in greater detail in Part IV.

CAMERA SUPPORT (TRIPOD)

The use of a tripod to eliminate camera shake is both a blessing and a detriment to medical photography (Fig. 44). Without question the sharpest image is created when the camera lens system is firmly fixed upon release of the shutter. In studios and offices where a relatively small volume of photography occurs, the use of a tripod is recommended, along with a cable release cord (Fig. 45) to further diminish any camera shake. Since the variety and design of tripods is virtually limitless, one should acquire a tripod unit with high flexibility for rapid changing of camera positions, light enough to move easily but sturdy enough to support whatever camera lens system is chosen. In particular, raising and

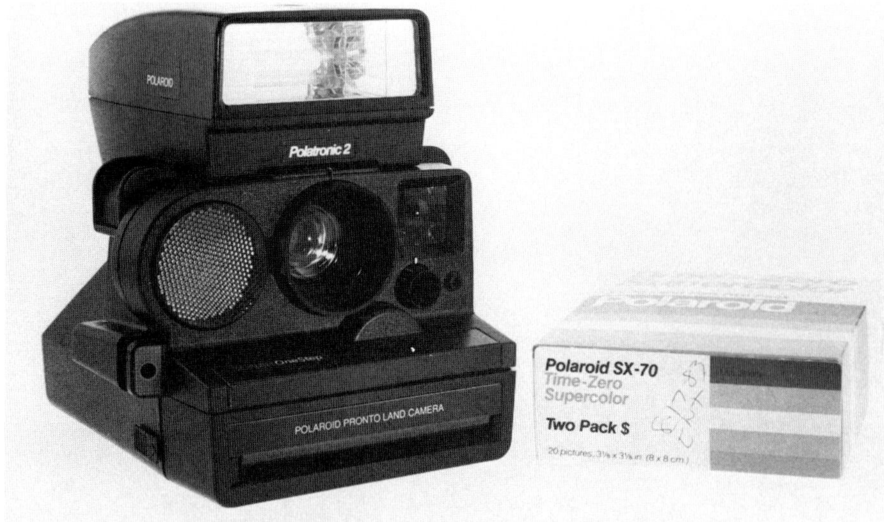

Figure 41. Standard Polaroid camera with limited focusing ability. More expensive Polaroid units are available, designed by specialty photography houses, which will interface with certain (but not all) SLR cameras. The latter units, although inordinately expensive, possess the advantages of utilization of 105 mm portrait lenses.

lowering the tripod quickly and easily is of prime importance in eliminating time delays during shooting.

In studios and offices where an enormous amount of photographic recording is carried out daily, the tripod becomes an impediment rather than an aid.

With care in camera stabilization, perfectly sharp photographs may be obtained by hand-holding the camera, avoiding the delays required for constant repositioning of the level and attitude of the camera-tripod complex. This is possible because of the relatively high shutter speed (1/125th of a second or more) combined with remarkably fast electronic flash bursts. The freedom to move about with the camera in office photography is a clear benefit and distinct timesaver, particularly under conditions in which unusual or nonroutine views are required (lacerations, scars, tumors, skin lesions).

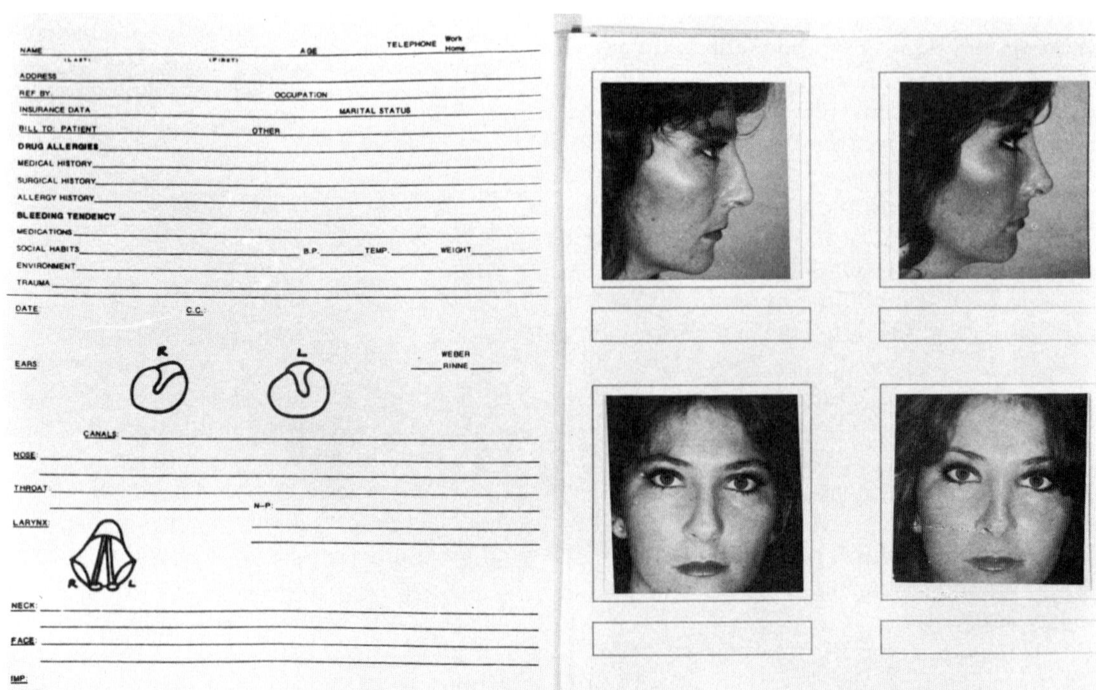

Figure 42. Polaroid print copies of accurate 2 × 2 slides filed in the patient's medical record for rapid and convenient evaluation.

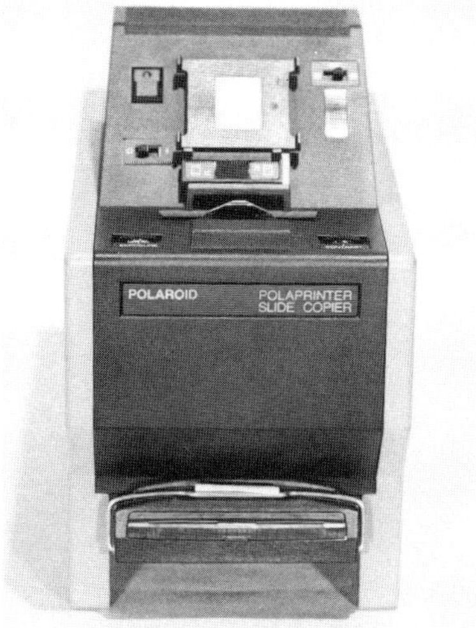

Figure 43. A convenient method of obtaining Polaroid color prints rapidly is by copying color slides with the use of the Polaprinter or Vivitar slide-to-print copier. This near foolproof method will provide, in minutes, excellent print copies of slides that will then be of uniform and standard size and illumination.

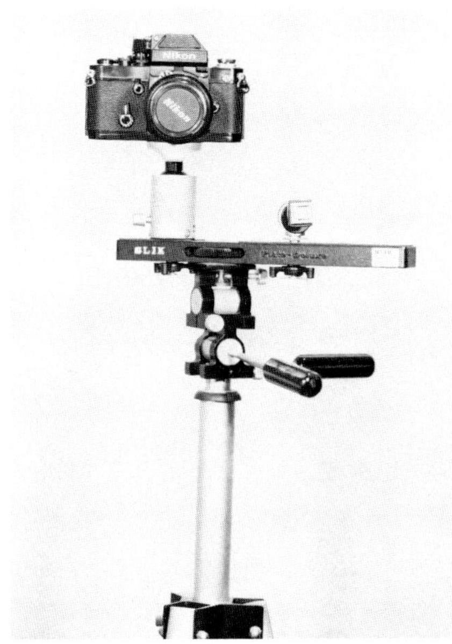

Figure 44. When time is of no consequence, use of the tripod to impart total immobility to the camera body is ideal. In copy work, such stabilization is essential. For routine patient photography, if care is taken, hand-holding the camera is both a more rapid and satisfactory method of obtaining the recommended head views quickly and efficiently.

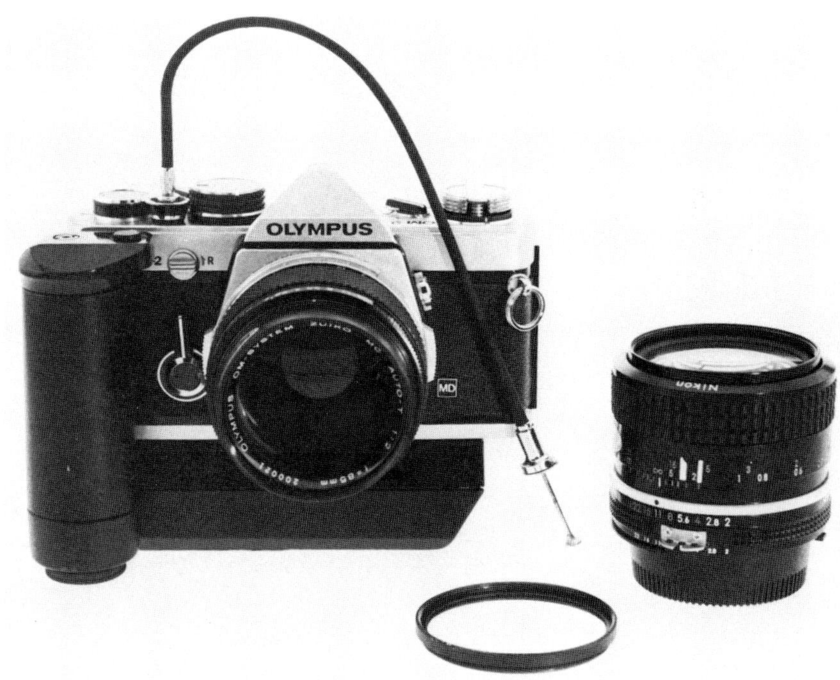

Figure 45. Typical cable release cord.

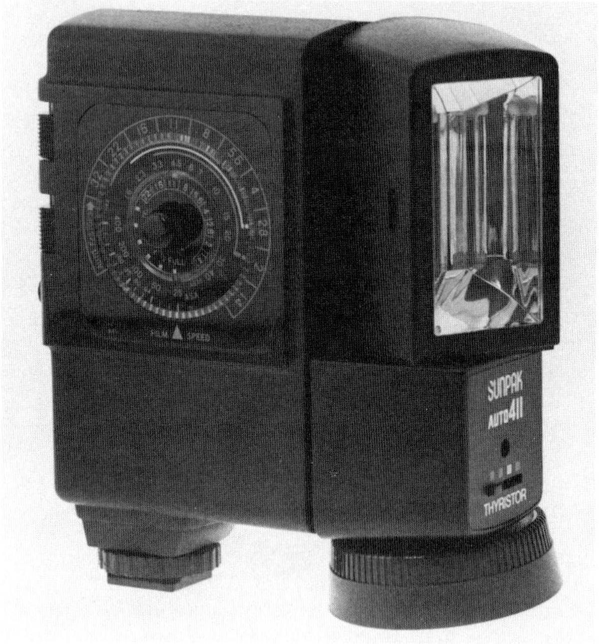

a

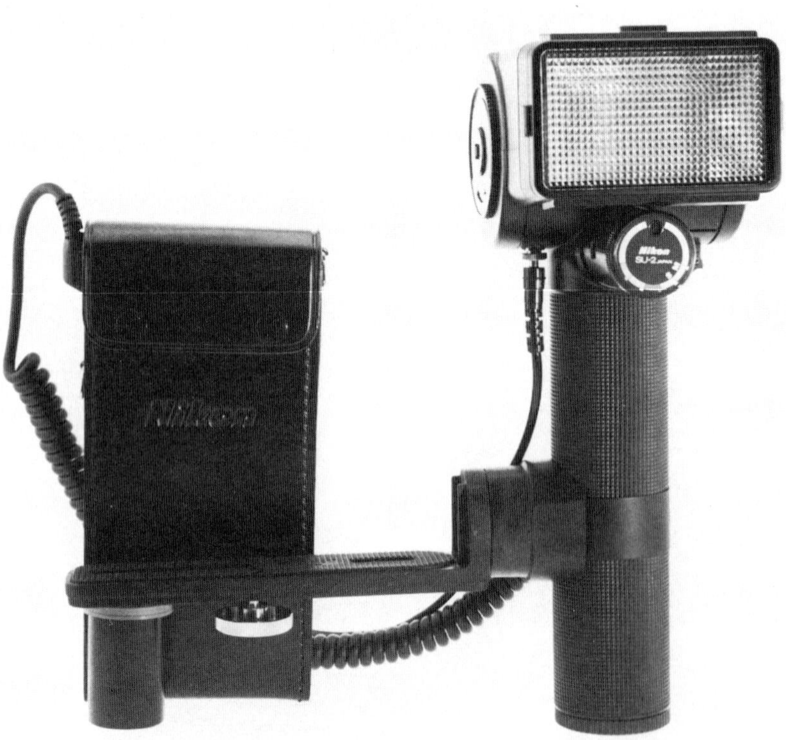

b

Figure 46. a,b, Small electronic flash units.

3 Lighting

ELECTRONIC LIGHTING

With the possible exception of faulty patient positioning, inaccurate lighting is the most common error encountered in medical photography. A brief review of any current journal relating to facial surgery will reflect this inadequacy, revealing photographic prints in overexposed, underexposed, and poorly modeled modes. To some degree this is surprising, since with only a minimum of effort lighting of extraordinarily high quality and uniformity can be achieved.

In the past decade one of the major advances in photography has been the development of remarkably powerful, lightweight, and relatively inexpensive electronic flash units (Fig. 46a-b). Since the control of light is perhaps the most critical challenge in creating an accurate image, electronic flash has simplified indoor photography as never before. A spin-off from space-age technology, compact flash units are sources of enormous energy controlled by miniaturized microcircuitry. With the possible exception of daylight, no other lighting provides such clean and natural lighting. With these tools at hand, then, superior medical photographs should be simpler than ever to create.

Electronic flash units are an exceptionally good value, since even the smallest, least complex units will provide many thousands of flash bursts, creating a remarkable savings over the conventional use of flash bulbs. Flash units containing "thyristor circuits" prevent surplus energy from the flash unit from reaching the flashtube, thereby conserving the power expended by each individual flash burst and shortening the recycle time for the capacitor to become fully recharged.

The basis for the system by which correct flash exposures are made is referred to as the "Inverse Square Law," a physical property of light that is familiar to all physicians:

> "The intensity of the light decreases as the square of the distance between light source and subject increases."

This law defines the constant relationship between *distance* and *illumination level.* A simple appreciation for this physical law will allow the medical photographer to understand more fully the setting of ideal and uniform lighting levels and to be able to compensate quickly when any additional variable is introduced.

In practical terms, then, if a light source positioned in front of the subject, e.g., 2 feet, is moved to 4 feet from the subject, the light falling on the subject will not be halved, but will decrease as the square of the distance (4^2 is 16). The photographer compensates for this dramatic fall-off in incident light by widening the aperture of the camera. Therefore, we can see that to expose any photograph properly, a predetermined balance between the *distance* and *aperture* setting needs to be established. To apply this theorem, it is necessary to appreciate that when the aperture (f-stop) is opened one stop, the amount of light entering the camera doubles, and closing the aperture one stop halves the amount of light allowed to enter.

In facial surgery in particular, the camera and electronic flash are ordinarily used in two fundamental ways. The first and most frequent use involves the recording of standard and uniform pre- and postoperative pictures for analysis, recordkeeping, and medicolegal documentation. Fortunately, once the proper set-up is arranged for these repetitive photographs, the photographer simply needs to follow the exact same protocol from sitting to sitting in order to ensure that the recorded images are uniform. The development of such a simple protocol is discussed later in this chapter.

The second major need for good photography in facial surgery involves the precise recording of surgical procedures in the operating room and the photography of small objects (specimens, foreign bodies, implants). The latter need demands a more exacting protocol, since many more variables are involved than in the relatively simple portrait photography used for uniform pre- and postoperative photography.

To ensure uniformly high-quality photographs in this nonuniform setting, one must take into consid-

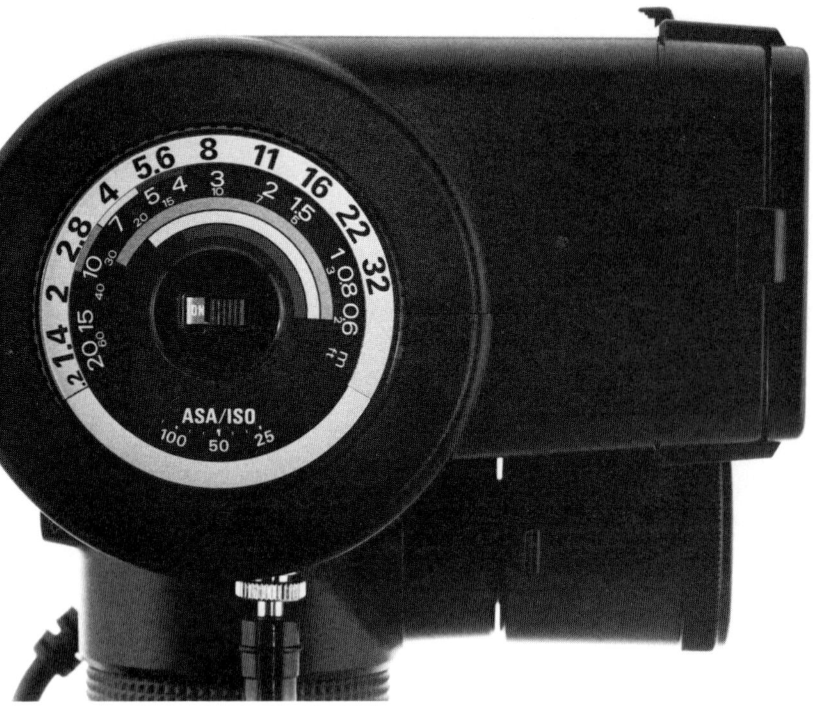

Figure 47. Calculator dial of a small electronic flash unit.

eration several additional variables, such as surrounding backgrounds, reflectivity of the photographed field or object, the varying distances of the object or objects from the flash unit, and other less controllable factors. To accomplish this, one must rely on the *Guide Number* of the flash unit being used. Since a significant difference may exist between the manufacturer's stated guide number and the true guide number, it is recommended that any new electronic flash unit be tested under varying conditions, keeping records, in order to establish the true characteristics for that particular flash unit.

To use the guide number properly and easily in facial photography, its derivation must be understood. Having established the manner in which distance correlates with f-stop numbers, we can now evaluate this relationship from the standpoint of maintaining constant ideal exposure when the subject-to-flash distance changes (such as in operative photography). Most small portable electronic flash units feature a calculator dial to assist the photographer in rapid computation of the correct f-stop for the flash-to-object distance (Fig. 47). To find the manufacturer's recommended guide number for any particular flash unit, simply multiply each f-number on the scale by its corresponding footage value (for example, f/4 × 16 feet, f/8 × 8 feet, f/11 × 5½ feet, f/16 × 4 feet); the result is approximately the same for every combination on the scale—around 64, the guide number for that particular unit. Any guide number may be determined by applying the formula:

> GUIDE NUMBER = DISTANCE (for correct exposure) × F-STOP (for correct exposure).

In any photographic situation, then, the proper f-stop can be determined by applying the formula in slightly different form:

> F-STOP = GUIDE NUMBER ÷ DISTANCE (flash to subject)

Thus, if your flash-to-subject distance is 20 feet, and the flash has a true guide number of 80, you would select f/4 for the correct exposure (f/4 = 80/20).

Since manufacturers may occasionally overstate their product's true guide numbers, it is wise to run some simple initial tests with your particular flash unit to ascertain the true guide number. A simple and rapid method of accomplishing this is to expose a series of test shots at different f-stops in the operating room (or in a simulated operating theater)

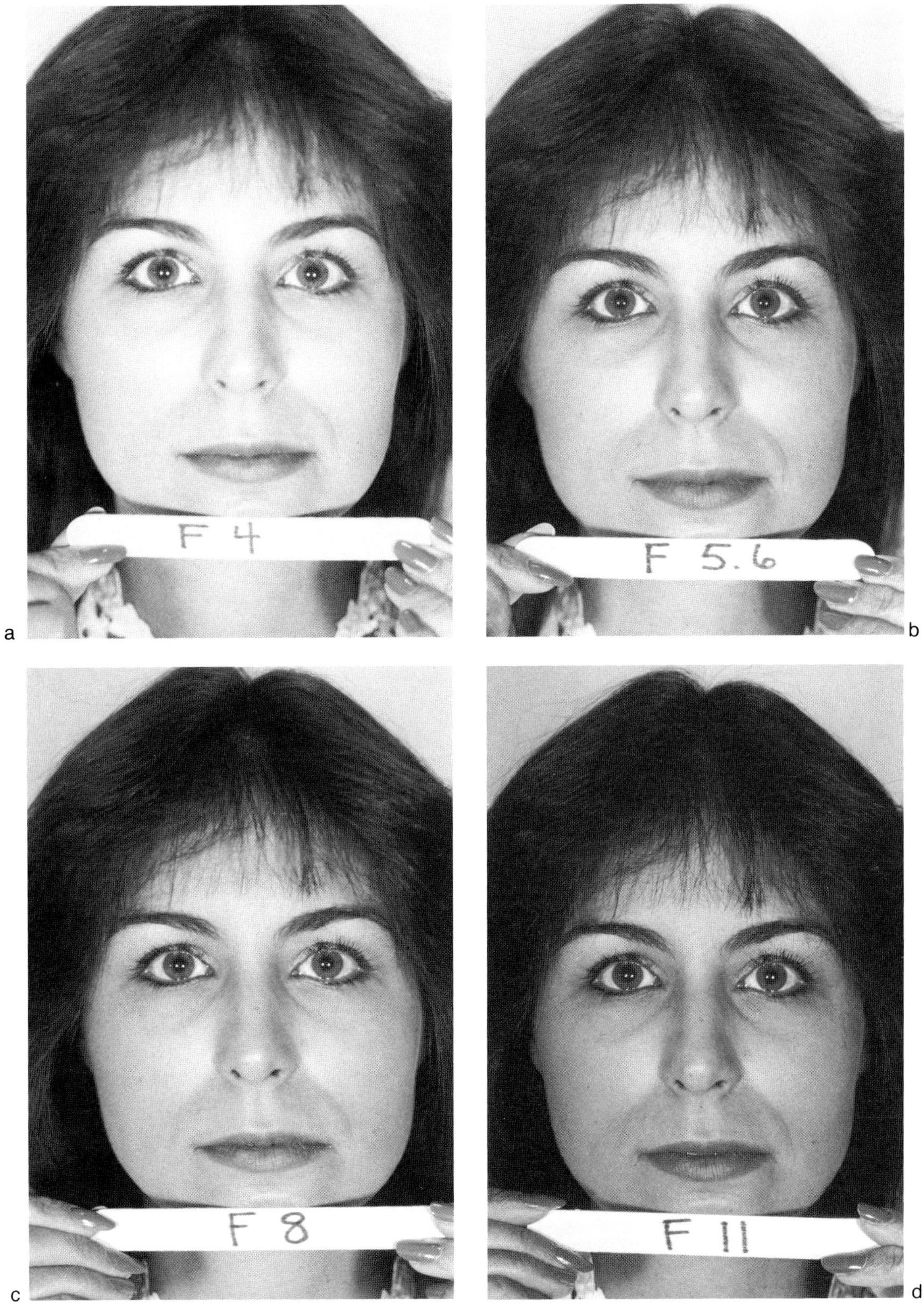

Figure 48. a–j, By exposing a series of shots at varying f-stops, with the distance and lighting remaining constant, the true guide number of any electronic flash may be rapidly and simply calculated. The ideal exposures, determined under actual working conditions, are then recorded on the flash dial for future reference. This sequence can be easily repeated at varying distances to predict accurately the correct f-stop for exact exposure.

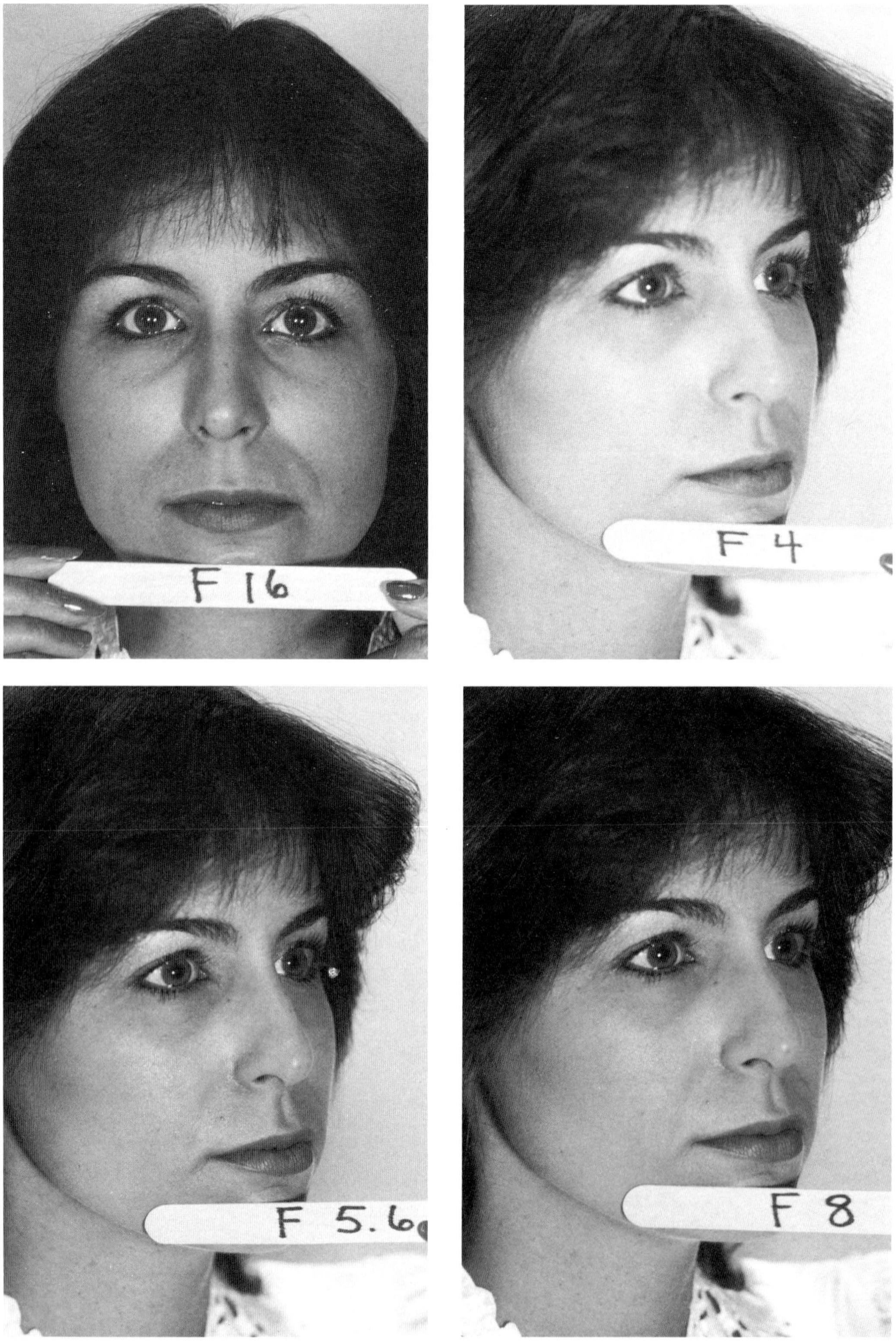

e f g h

Figure 48. *(Continued)*

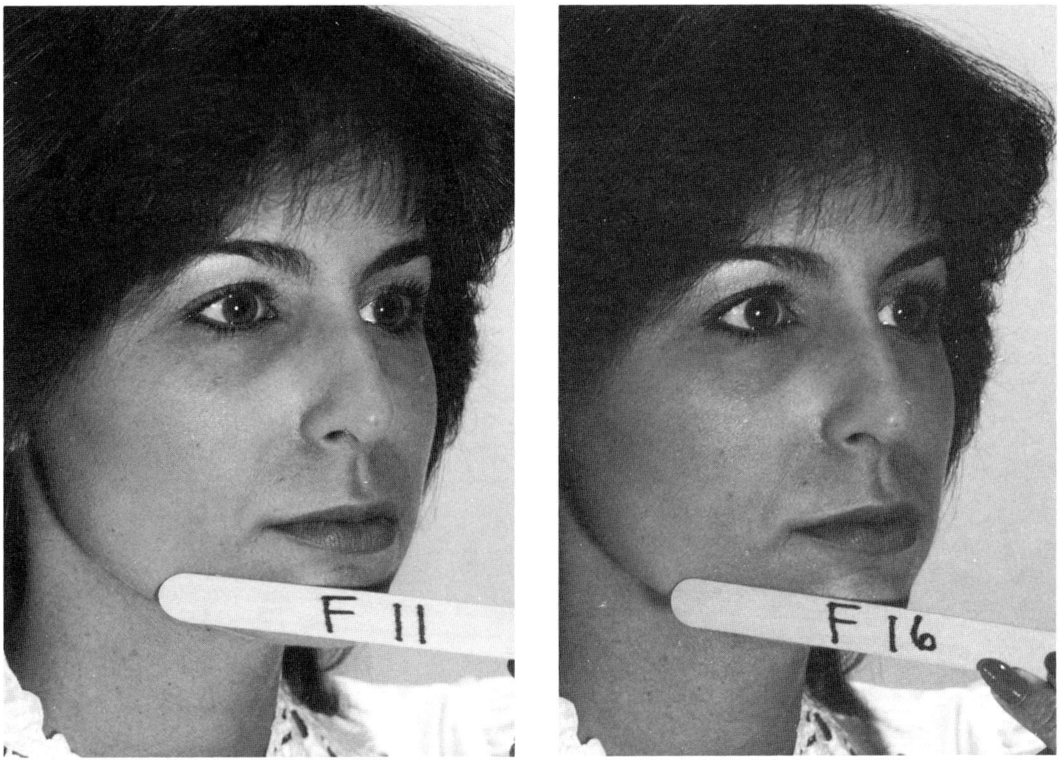

i j

Figure 48. *(Continued)*

(Fig. 48a-j). By marking each consecutive f-stop on a tongue blade placed in the field to be photographed, and exposing each test shot at exactly the same distance, the best f-stop exposure for your needs may be easily selected after the film is processed. We recommend using only Kodachrome 25 or 64 for this comparison test. By applying the formula, the true guide number for your individual flash unit can be easily and quickly (and confidently) selected.

Remember that compensations for varying conditions must be regularly made, involving one-half to one whole stop compensations. When photographing black skin, a dark field, a bloody field, or a field surrounded by very dark surgical drapes, one may wish to open the aperture one-half to one f-stop. If conditions of extremely light shiny skin, highly reflective surfaces, or very light surgical drapes exist, the image exposure may be improved by closing the aperture one-half to one stop.

Finally, of course, all good medical photographers ensure that proper exposures will be regularly obtained by intentionally "bracketing" (exposing the shot one-half to one stop above and below the recommended aperture setting) during important photographic sessions (Fig. 49a-c). Since conditions and anatomy change from moment to moment in surgery, only one fleeting opportunity may present itself to record an all-important event.

Two major factors should influence the selection of an electronic flash unit: the *guide number* and the *recycle time*. Higher guide numbers assigned to small on-camera flash units generally reflect a more powerful unit capable of emitting more energy in each light burst. This allows you shooting with smaller apertures to increase the depth of field, a desirable feature. Particularly in operative surgical situations, where time and speed are factors, units with more rapid recycle times are valuable. It is wise to remember that most recycle ready lights glow at slightly less than full charge, which means that exposures made the instant the light glows may well be underexposed. At least 2 seconds should elapse after the ready light glows before releasing the shutter. The use of AC adaptor power or more powerful rechargeable nickel-cadmium battery packs can speed the recycle times and allow more rapid exposures.

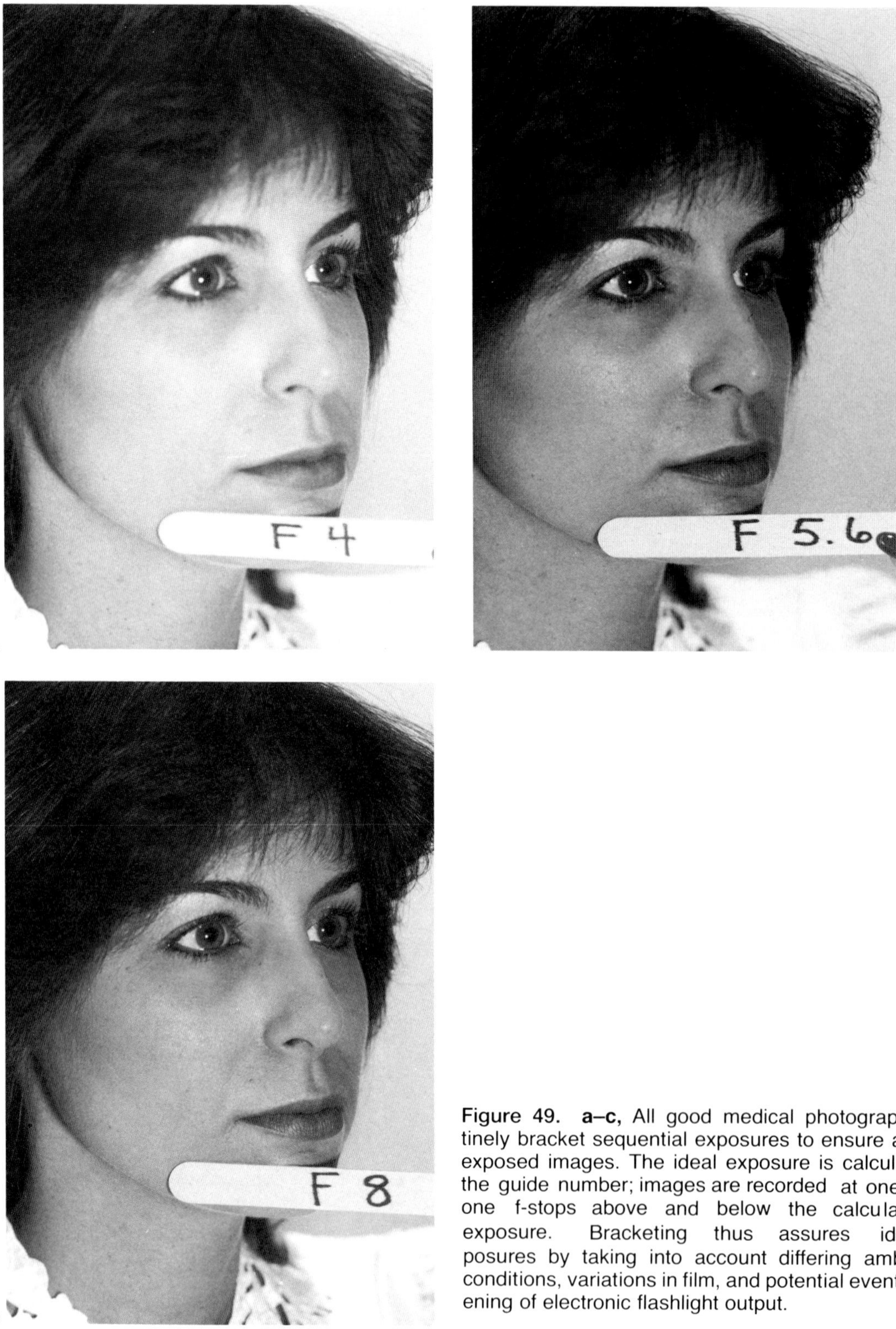

a b c

Figure 49. **a–c,** All good medical photographers routinely bracket sequential exposures to ensure accurately exposed images. The ideal exposure is calculated from the guide number; images are recorded at one-half and one f-stops above and below the calculated ideal exposure. Bracketing thus assures ideal exposures by taking into account differing ambient light conditions, variations in film, and potential eventual weakening of electronic flashlight output.

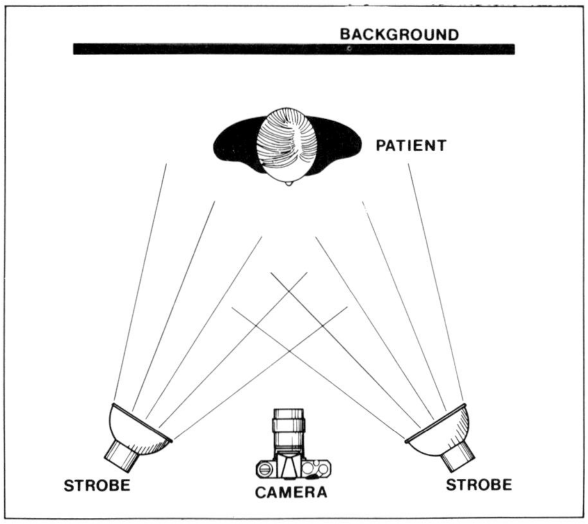

Figure 50. Dual studio electronic flash units, reflected and diffused by large umbrellas, remain the ideal light source for excellent lighting of patient subjects.

DUAL ELECTRONIC FLASH UNITS

The best portrait photographs are consistently made utilizing dual electronic flash units positioned on either side of the camera, synchronized to fire simultaneously when triggered by the camera shutter release. The distance from the camera of each flash strobe unit is again a matter of personal taste, but in order to achieve uniform facial lighting without casting asymmetric modeling shadows (an interesting but medically inaccurate effect), the flash heads should be approximately the same distance from the camera, and at nearly the same level as the camera. In this manner uniform lighting can be achieved from session to session with the same patient, making it easy to compare serial photographs accurately.

Preventing harsh background shadows is accomplished quite simply in the following fashion. First, the patient should be moved sufficiently forward of the background so that harsh shadows are significantly softened. Within the limits of space and comfort, positioning the patient at least 2 feet from the background will accomplish this goal. If diffusing screens or umbrellas are used on the individual flash heads to soften and diffuse the incident light, less severe shadows will result.

Although acceptable portrait facial images can be made using a single electronic flash unit positioned on the camera body itself, this on-camera flash technique produces a characteristically flat, two-dimensional effect, with harsh highlights and washed-out skin tones as typical side effects. In addition, unacceptable and unnecessary shadows are almost always cast on the background by the single on-camera flash, and, therefore, we recommend its use only when the dual flash system is not available, or in emergencies.

Optimal patient photography then requires the use of studio grade electronic flash units, positioned in some fashion on either side of the camera (Fig. 50). Although excellent results can be obtained with two small portable electronic flash units mounted on a bracket on either side of the camera (Fig. 51), versatility and power are lost in this arrangement. Our preference and recommendation then is to choose a small studio-type electronic flash set-up that occupies little space in the medical office (Fig. 52), is capable of powerful bursts of light output, allowing smaller aperture settings (and therefore greater potential depth of field), and provides superb modeling capability to capture in great detail the precise form of the human face.

Such an arrangement requires a slightly greater investment of money at the outset, but this drawback is more than offset by the great volume of flash bursts available (ordinarily more than 50,000) and the remarkable quality provided with Kodak slow-speed, fine-grain films (Kodachrome 25 and 64). In addition, the dual electronic studio flash units, because of their remarkable power output, allow the photographer to use indirect, diffused, or softened light to eliminate bright spots and harsh highlights to produce the very best image.

A recommended arrangement for dual studio flash units is illustrated in Figure 53. The two flash units are positioned on either side of the camera at approximately the same distance from the subject. Mounted on lightweight aluminum telescoping stands, their position and height can be easily and quickly adjusted according to the patient's height and individual needs. Connected to the camera body by synchronized cords, the units fire simultaneously when the shutter is released, being controlled by a central power pack.

Second, employing an overhead "kicker" or "key" light (Fig. 54), positioned on the ceiling and activated by a remote "slave" device, will illuminate the background, effectively eliminating any potential shadows and adding a backlighting effect that further improves the picture quality and creates a near three-dimensional effect. These remote slave units are quite inexpensive, and even are produced as self-contained screw-in strobe bulbs.

Many studio strobe flash units are provided with a so-called "modeling" light mounted near or within the strobe unit, consisting of a weak, continuous light source. The modeling lights allow an assessment of the effect the placement of the dual strobe units will have on the ultimate image recorded, and in imperfectly lit rooms, allow improved focusing before exposing the image.

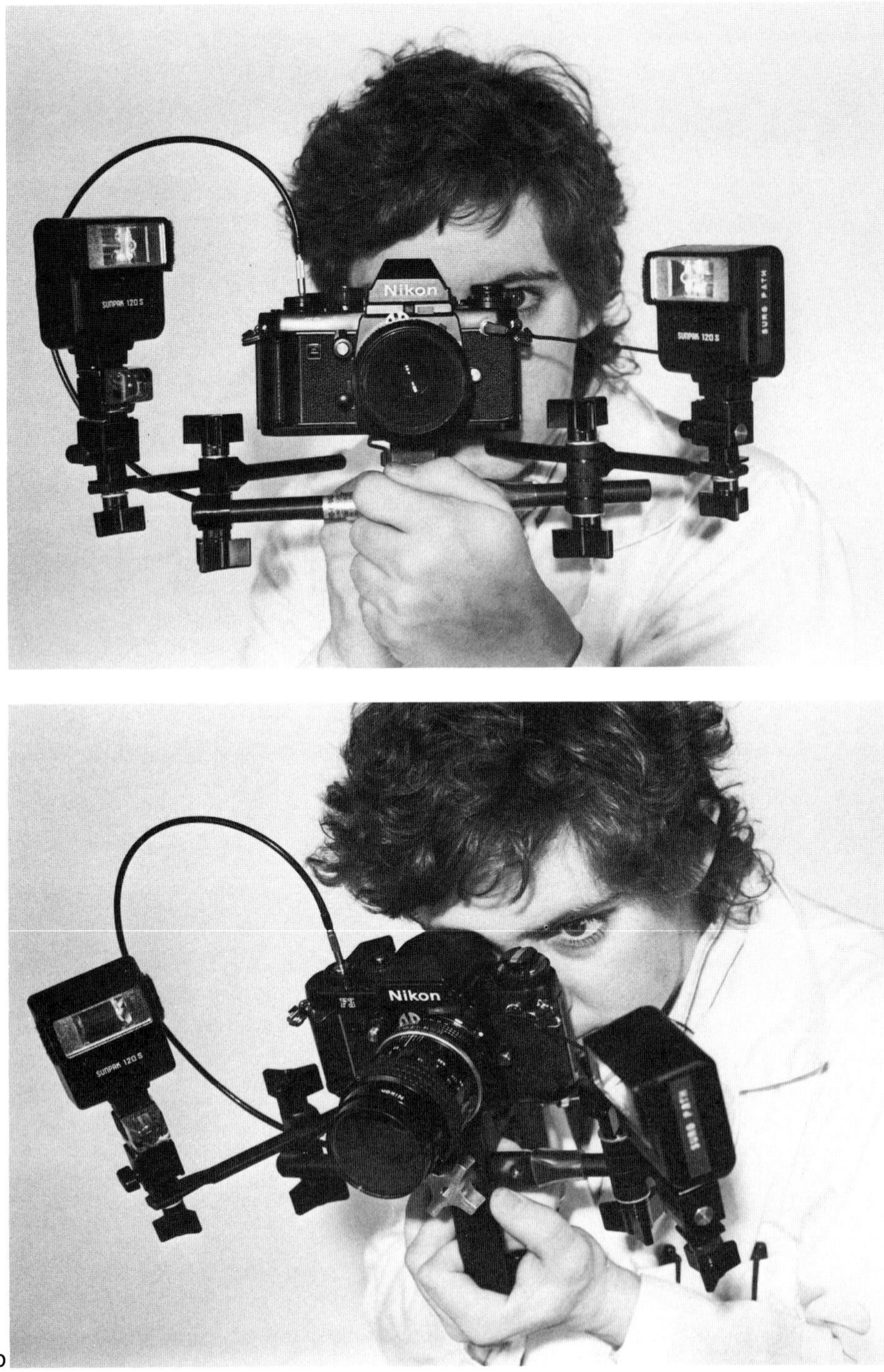

a b

Figure 51. a,b, Brackets are commercially available to support the camera body and dual compact electronic flash units. Although these arrangements may often result in superb images being recorded, the units are somewhat unwieldy and impractical for offices in which a large volume of photography is carried out.

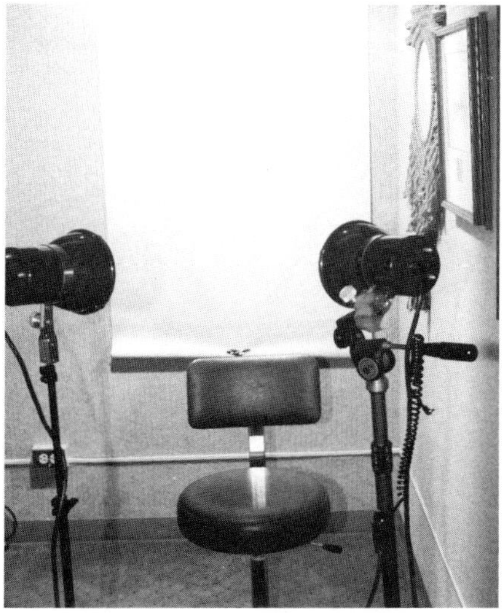

Figure 52. Compact dual studio-style electronic flash units are an ideal arrangement for office photography, requiring little space while delivering many thousands of uniform electronic flash bursts. We recommend them for use by the office surgeon-photographer.

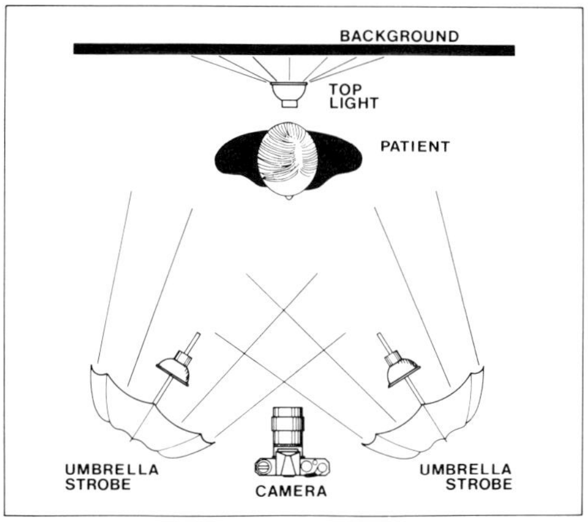

Figure 53. One recommended arrangement for office positioning of camera, patient, and dual electronic flash units.

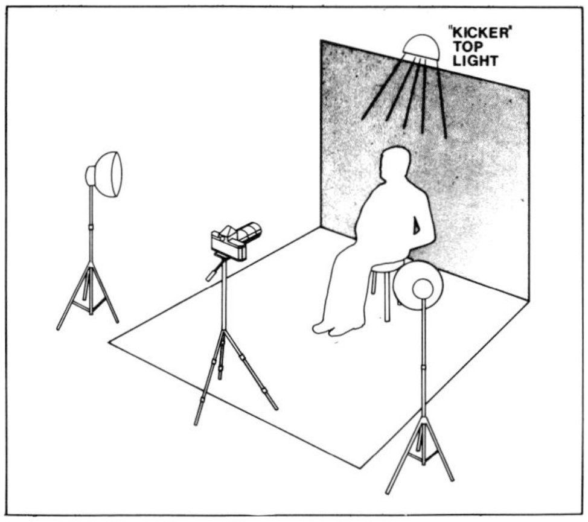

Figure 54. Overhead "key" or "kicker" lights soften or eliminate background shadows and serve to highlight the patient's head and hair, providing one more ingredient of a simulated three-dimensional effect.

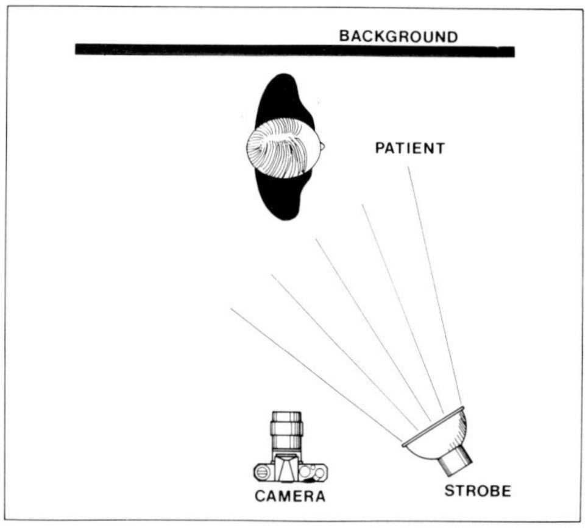

Figure 55. Recommended positioning and alignment for recording right lateral view. One or both strobe lights may be used.

Once the dual electronic strobe units have been positioned to your satisfaction, it is mandatory to perform the simple but critical sample exposure tests, the same ones described with the single on-camera flash unit in the operating room.

A subject with average skin tones is seated on the rotating stool or chair in front of the background, and the face and head are positioned in the frontal plane. A series of test shots is then recorded with the patient holding a small 3 by 5 card (or tongue blade) on which has been recorded the f-stop for that particular shot (see Fig. 48). Sample shots are made in the lateral and oblique positions as well, since one may wish to use slightly different lighting in these positions (this, of course, implies that the lighting differences will be carried forth for all future photographs of that same patient for complete standardization (Figs. 55-58). Selecting the best exposure from this test series will now be a simple matter for the surgeon, and that setting can henceforth be used to maintain complete uniformity of lighting and exposure from sitting to sitting.

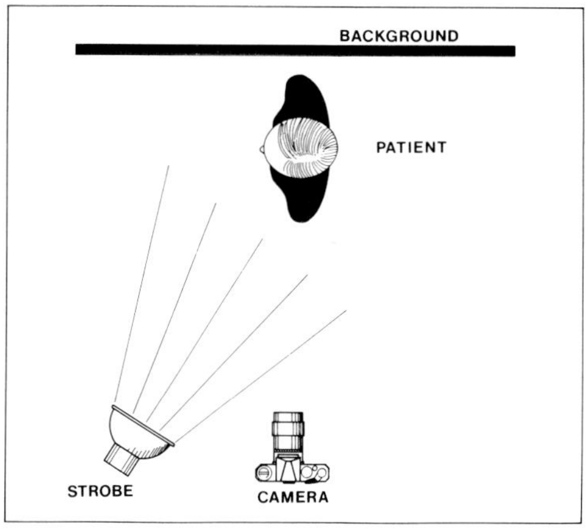

Figure 56. Recommended positioning and alignment for recording left lateral view.

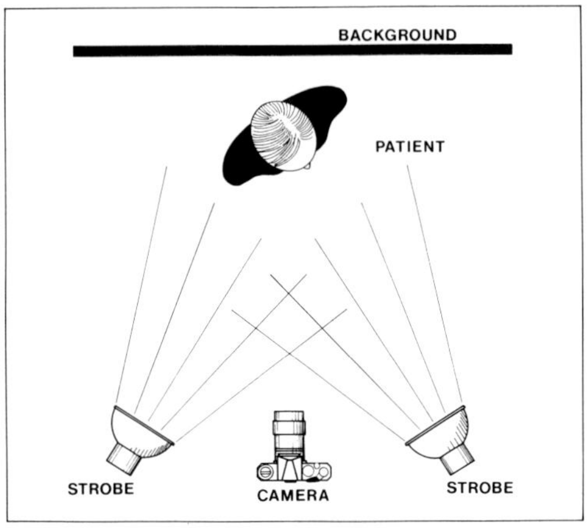

Figure 57. Positioning for right oblique view.

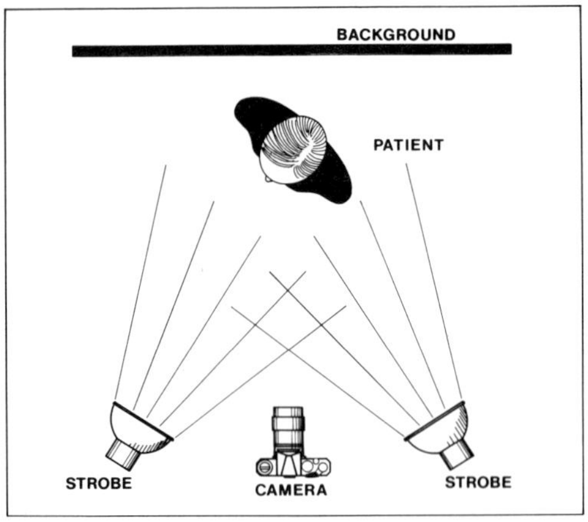

Figure 58. Positioning for left oblique view.

It should be appreciated that all variables have been eliminated except for patient positioning, probably the most commonly inaccurate factor in uniform photography. The photographer must constantly be on guard for minor variations in patient positioning and correct them before the image is exposed.

RING FLASH UNITS

Since they have achieved some popularity in the past decade in medical photography, a comment should be made about the use of ring flash units in facial photography (Fig. 59). Since it surrounds the lens, the ring flash provides completely frontal, shadowless lighting; that is, all of the shadows created fall directly behind the subject or object to be photographed. For that reason, it would seem to eliminate one of the unpleasant variables inherent in facial photography and simplify the task of recording a near-perfect image. This, indeed, holds true for small object and specimen photography. Unfortunately, its advantages are lost in facial portrait photography, in which the uniform modeling and detailing characteristics created by dual strobe units are not only pleasing, but useful in assessing facial asymmetry and feature relationships. The

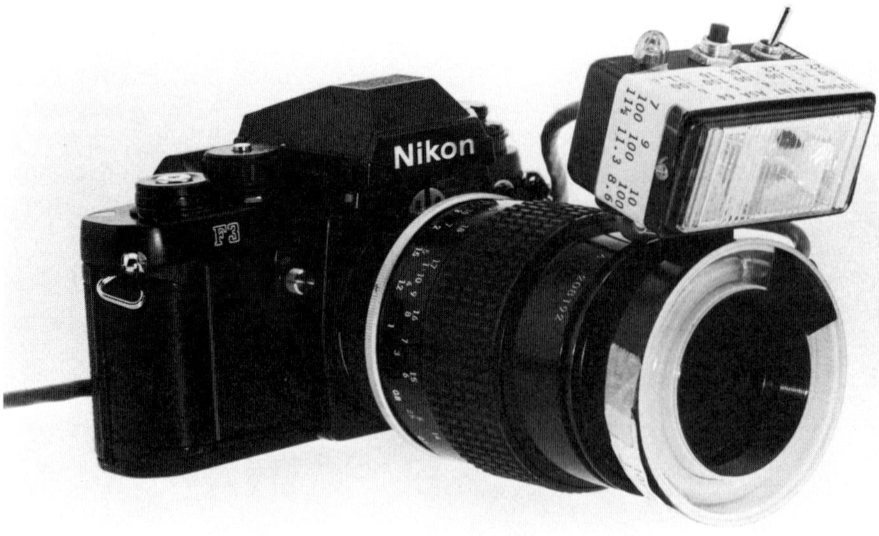

Figure 59. One form of ring flash with attached point light to increase modeling effect. Ring flash illumination is ideal for all intracavitary photography to achieve near shadowless lighting; in facial portrait photography the image produced is too often flat, harsh, and without the important modeling effect obtained with balanced dual flash units.

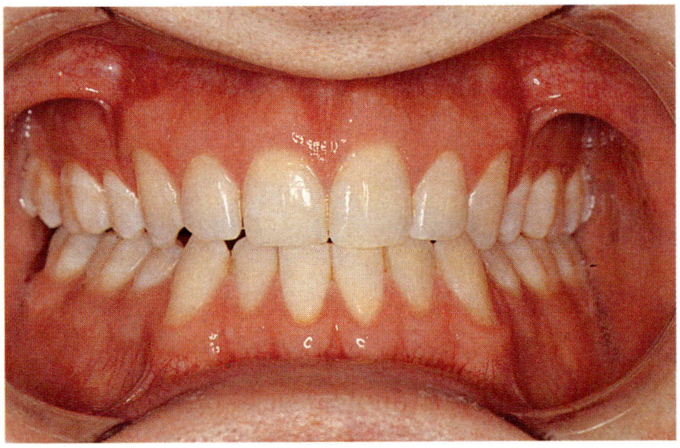

Figure 60. Intraoral photograph obtained with ring flash illumination. Note even and balanced lighting with the elimination of most shadows.

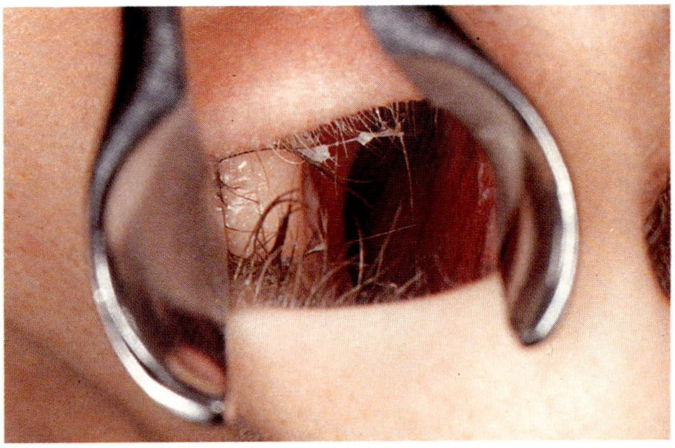

Figure 61. Intranasal photographs are facilitated with the use of the ring flash, since the intranasal regions are difficult to illuminate properly and completely with conventional flash units.

flat, shadowless, and somewhat harsh image recorded by ring flash units is therefore decidedly inferior to the image recorded by nonring flash methods previously described. In addition, ring flash units tend to be considerably more expensive than more conventional on-camera strobe units, thereby limiting their usefulness.

Ring flash units are ideal and preferred for all *intracavitary* photography, where uniform shadowless lighting is otherwise difficult to achieve. In dentistry, intraoral photographs provided by ring flash units are superb (Fig. 60); the same principle holds true for intranasal (and other intracavitary) photographic needs (Fig. 61).

For the best results in facial photography, where the nuances of form, detail, and the suggestion of a third dimension are desirable, the lighting provided by ring flash units is clearly inferior.

From the foregoing suggestions, it can be seen that, as never before, the medical photographer has at his command a marvelous array of compact, powerful, lightweight, and relatively inexpensive electronic flash equipment from which to choose. Any number of brands and packaging descriptions will be capable of creating satisfactory and even outstanding photographs.

The key, however, is to select equipment that can be easily and repetitively used to procure standard and uniform images that are comparable in positioning, lighting, size, and color. The cost and brand name of strobe units are the least important factors in the quality of facial image portraits produced. What is critically important is to select recommended equipment that is satisfactorily used by others with experience, to establish with simple testing an easily repeatable system, and to reproduce that system faithfully from sitting to sitting for precise patient photography.

4 Guidelines for Specific Plastic Surgical Procedures

If the foregoing rules are followed, the vast majority of sequential patient photographs will demonstrate high uniformity and standardization. It is useful, then, to review a variety of common operations performed in head and neck plastic surgery, noting the positioning principles critical to the accurate photographic recording of each.

RHINOPLASTY

Six views are essential to evaluate and document the nasal appearance adequately before surgery. Optional additional views may be indicated and helpful in special circumstances.

Frontal View (Fig. 62a)

With the patient in repose, the head is aligned with the Frankfort horizontal line parallel to the floor. The head and the camera lens should be positioned on the same plane, with the patient looking directly into the lens. The midsagittal line should be positioned directly down the midline of the face, so that the head is accurately aligned, with equal amounts of the external ear apparent on either side.

Base View (Fig. 62b)

Next the head is lifted so that the tip of the nose is positioned precisely at the level of the eyebrows. Again, it is important that the midsagittal line be precisely midline, and that the horizontal plane of the face is parallel to the floor.

Right Lateral View (Fig. 62c)

The patient is now turned 90° so that positioning for the lateral view may be accomplished. With the hair pulled back and controlled with combs, pins, or elastic bands to expose the external ear, the head is positioned with the Frankfort horizontal line precisely parallel to the floor. The head should be positioned looking straight ahead with the eyes open. Accurate positioning may be facilitated when sighting through the camera by axially aligning the upper eyelashes or the lateral commissures of the oral cavity, or both. The patient's posture should be erect, leaning neither forward nor backward, since these positions tend to introduce a factor of distortion and misinformation.

Right Oblique View (Fig. 62d)

The patient is rotated 45° to the right, and the head is aligned so that a vertical line dropped from the right inner canthus will intersect the right oral commissure. The Frankfort horizontal line must be carefully aligned during this view, since patients tend to tilt the head inadvertently.

Left Lateral View (Fig. 62e)

Same alignment as right lateral view, except from the left.

Left Oblique View (Fig. 62f)

Same alignment as the right oblique view, except from the left.

Some surgeons prefer a lateral smiling view to demonstrate animation and anatomic alterations occurring when the patient smiles (Fig. 63). An estimate of the synergistic action of the nasal and facial mimetic muscles may be judged thereby.

Close-up views of the base of the nose are preferred by some to provide an enlargement of the nasal base, but these are not essential.

Frontal views of the twisted nose with a straight object (ruler or tongue blade) positioned in the midsagittal line will be helpful in documenting the asymmetries that exist (Fig. 64) and can be invaluable in facilitating understanding in the patient who has failed to recognize subtle and even more pro-

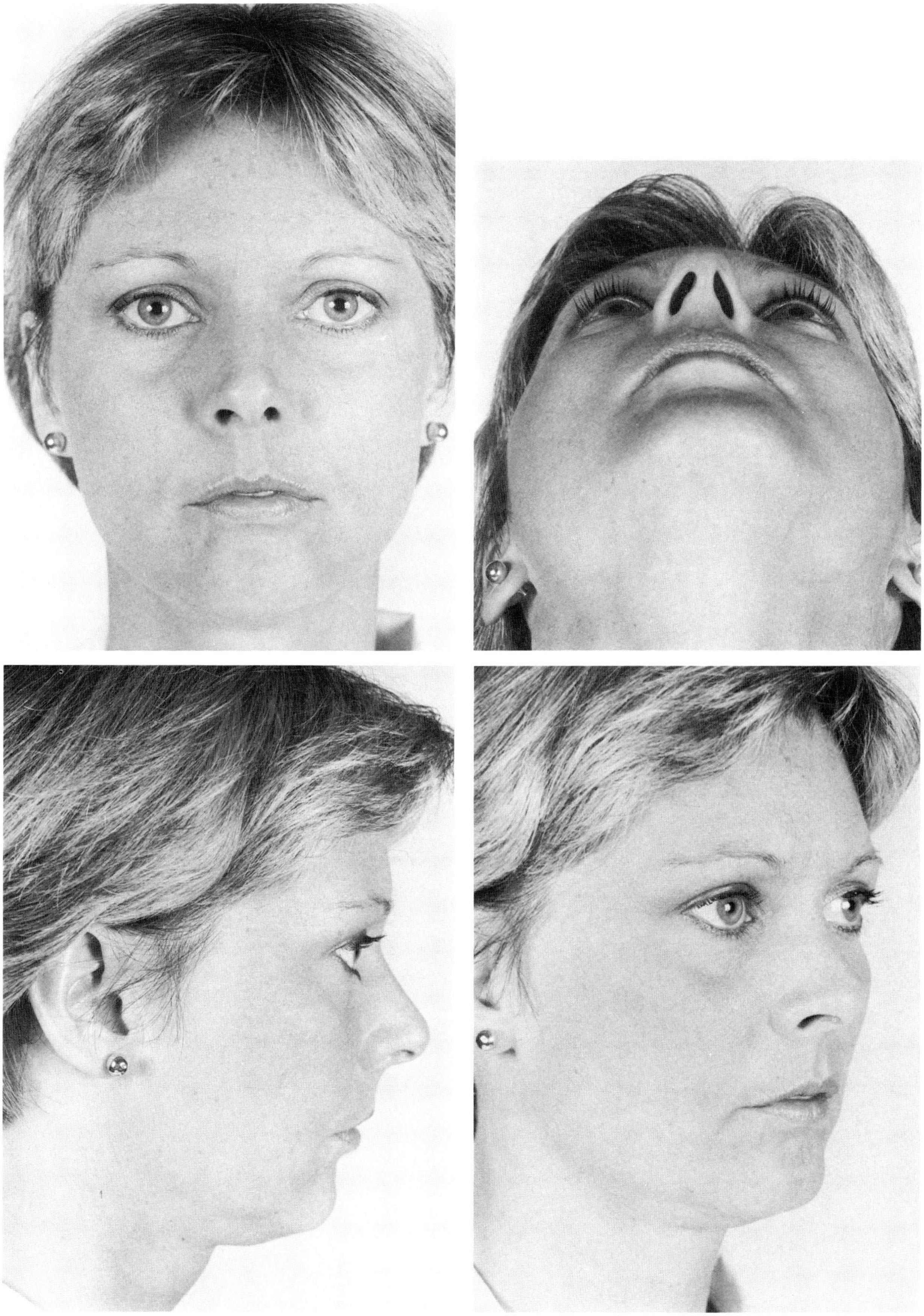

a b c d

Figure 62. **a–f,** Routine views of the nose in frontal, lateral, basal, and oblique positions are the minimum that should be obtained in all patients undergoing rhinoplasty. By following the positioning guidelines outlined in the text, standard and uniform views may be obtained from sitting to sitting for accurate comparison and documentation.

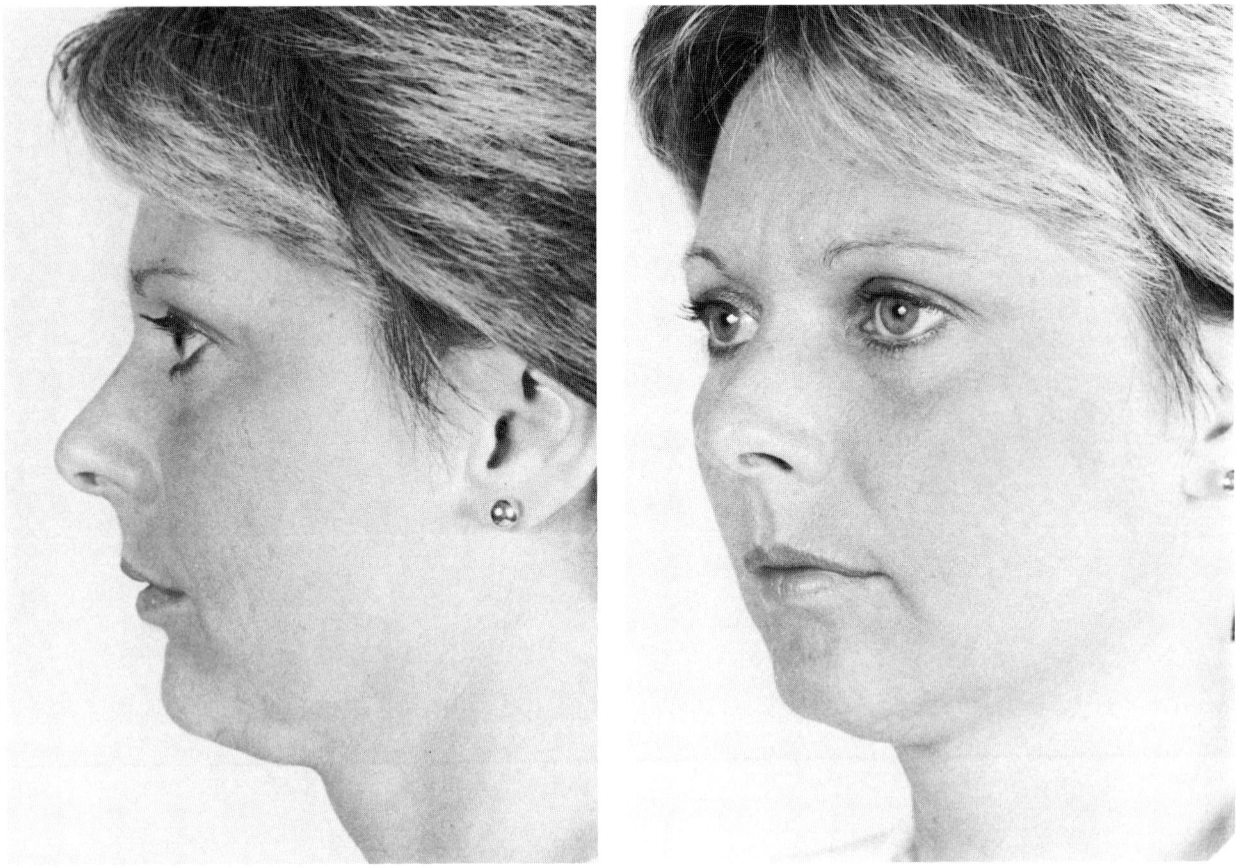

e f

Figure 62. *(Continued)*

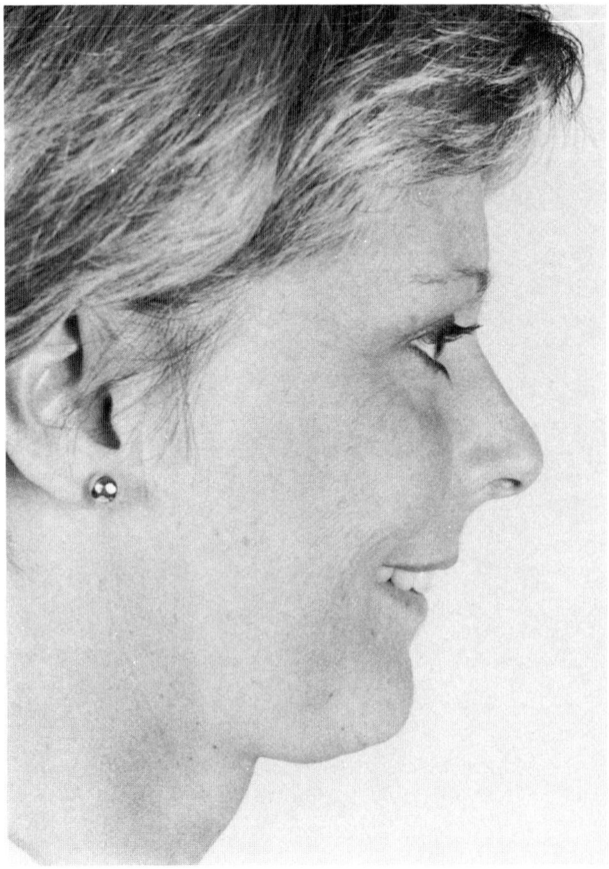

Figure 63. A smiling view, although optional, may provide important information regarding the dynamics of the nose and face upon animation and thereby aid the surgeon in preoperative planning.

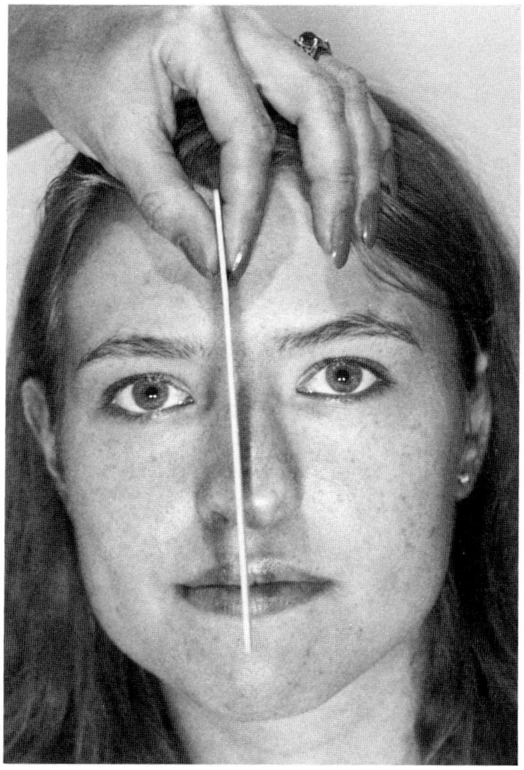

Figure 64. Some subtle twists of the nose may be more dramatically documented by photographing a straight object in the midline to emphasize imbalance and disproportion.

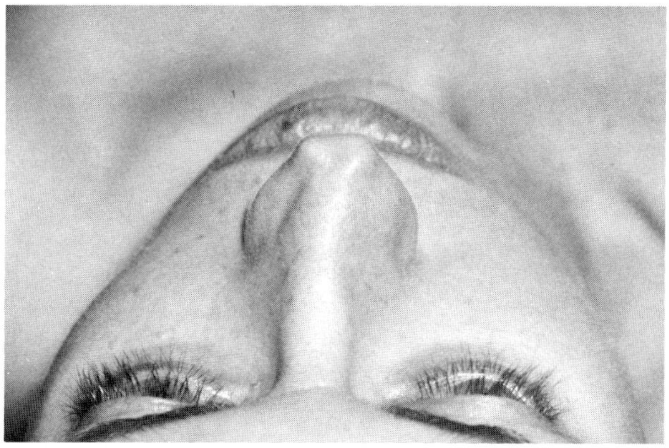

Figure 65. Photographs of the twisted nose taken from above downward may document more clearly the deviated nose, less well appreciated on routine frontal views.

found nasal deviations from the midline. Subtle deviations may also be documented with frontal views of the patient's face tilted downward, or with a view obtained from above and behind the head (Fig. 65).

BLEPHAROPLASTY

Six views are informative in documenting blepharoplastic surgery and may be helpful as well in all forms of periorbital surgical repair.

Frontal View—Eyes Open (Fig. 66a)

This view is identical to that taken for rhinoplasty, with the patient looking directly at the camera lens. Precise horizontal positioning is critical to prevent a spurious assessment of the relationship of the lower lid to the limbus pre- and postoperatively. Brow position is assessed in this view.

Frontal View—Eyes Closed (Fig. 66b)

With eyes closed in repose, the anatomy of the upper lid and infrabrow area is better evaluated. Complete upper lid closure (or lack of closure, as in facial paralysis or overzealous upper lid skin removal) is appreciated. The degree of upper lid pigmentation, an important factor in preoperative analysis, is best seen in this view.

Frontal View—Upward Gaze (Fig. 66c)

This view primarily accentuates the lower lid fat prominence and may help to delineate specific compartmentalization of orbital fat in preoperative planning.

Right Lateral View (Fig. 66d)

Lateral views demonstrate not only the degree of lower lid fat protrusion, they also help to delineate

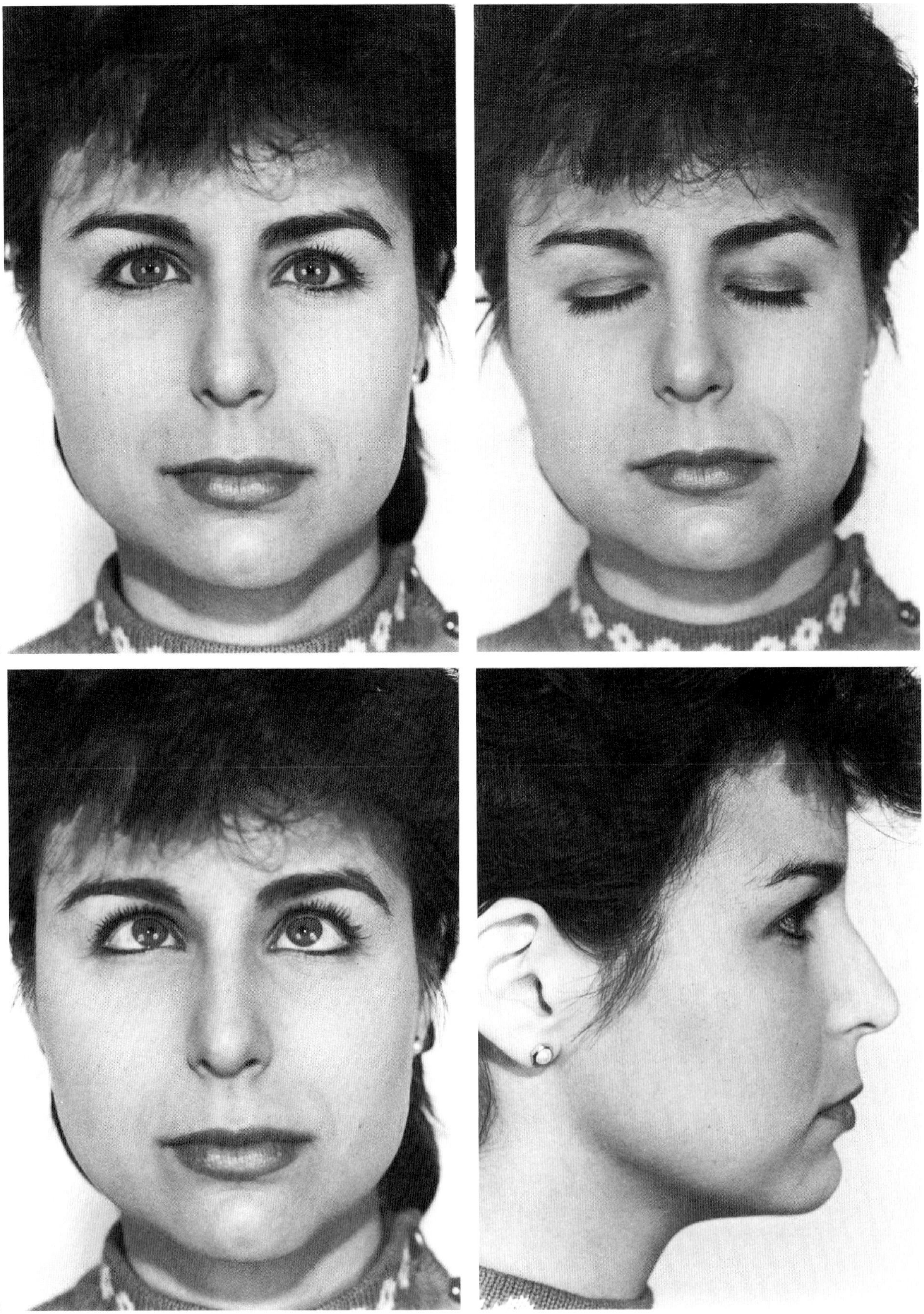

a b c d

Figure 66. a–f, Routine blepharoplasty and orbital trauma views.

creases and wrinkling adjacent to the lateral canthus, brow ptosis, and presence or absence of a satisfactory supratarsal cleft.

Left Lateral View (Fig. 66e)

Same alignment as right lateral view, except from the left.

Close-up Frontal View (Fig. 66f)

With the eyes open, a close-up view taken to include only the brows and nose flanking the orbits is helpful to demonstrate greater detail for planning. A close-up view with upward gaze is also useful to emphasize herniated lower lid fat.

Additional optional views include oblique three-quarter views of each eye, extreme close-ups of each orbit, and frontal views taken in all the directions of cardinal gaze. In unusual and specific situations, these optional orbital views may be helpful and even mandatory for precise documentation. After periorbital trauma, we routinely include these optional periorbital views.

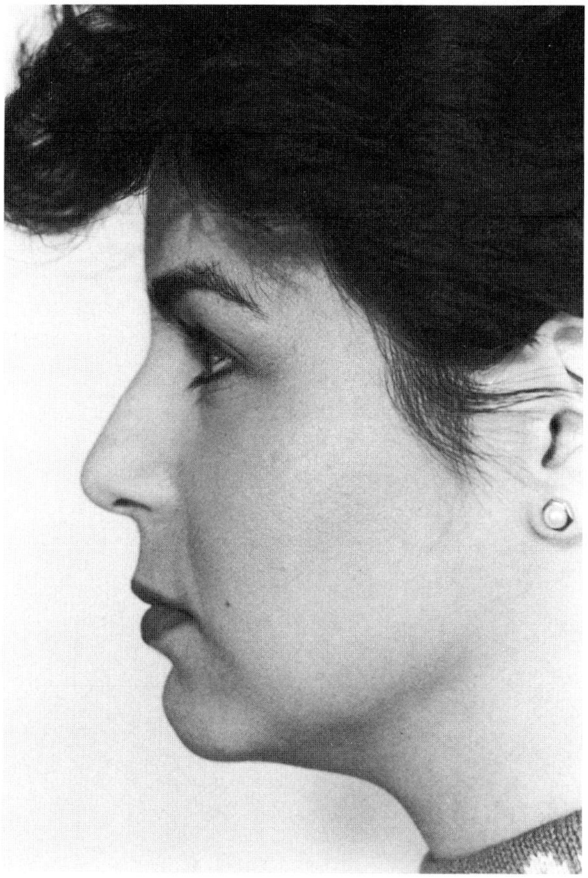

e

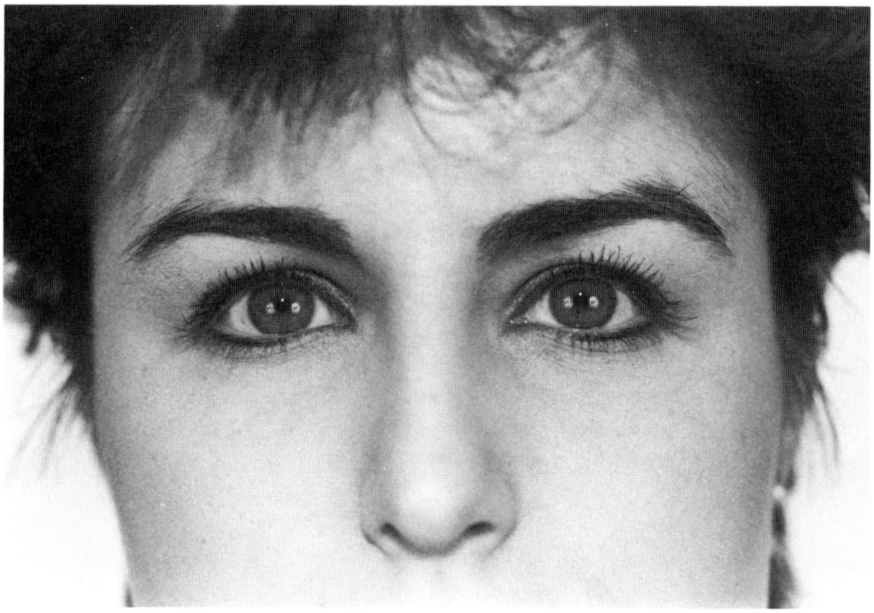

f

Figure 66. *(Continued)*

RHYTIDOPLASTY

Six views are recommended to document the patient's condition and appearance adequately. Unlike other facial surgery views, it is essential in rhytidoplasty photography to include the neck in the photographic image, since much of the improvement resulting from rhytidoplasty is reflected in the appearance of the neck. The six views are:

1. Frontal view—repose (Fig. 67a)
2. Frontal view—smiling (Fig. 67b)

3,4. Right and left oblique views (Fig. 67c,d)
5,6. Right and left lateral views (Fig. 67e,f)

An optional seventh view may be desired with the patient performing a marked contortional grimace (Fig. 68a,b), documenting the action and position of the mimetic muscles and their action on facial and cervical appearance. In particular, forcibly contracting the platysma muscle bands allows documentation of the free edges of the platysma and may help in planning for repositioning or recontouring the muscle during corrective face and neck surgery.

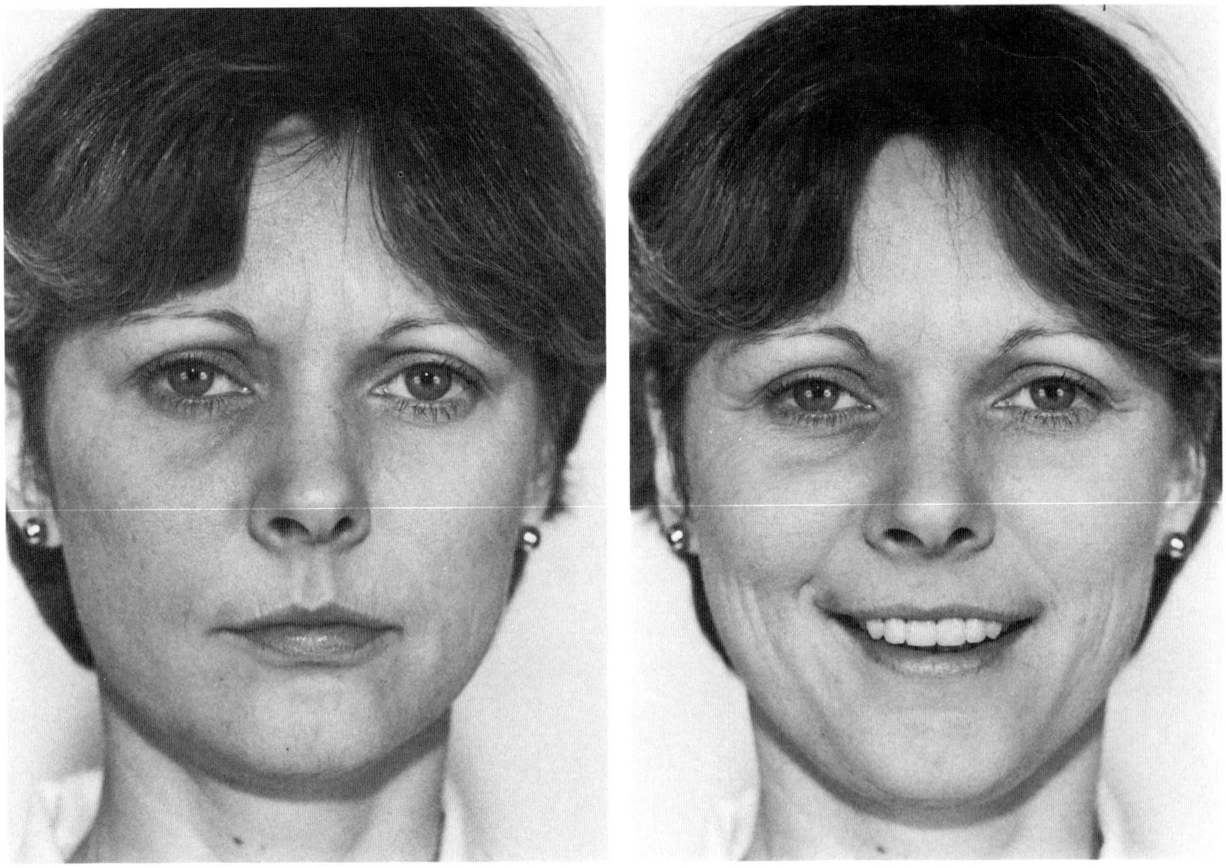

a b

Figure 67. a–f, Routine rhytidoplasty views. Unlike facial photographs for other conditions, views of the rhytidoplasty patient should include the neck area to document cervical abnormalities as well as improvements.

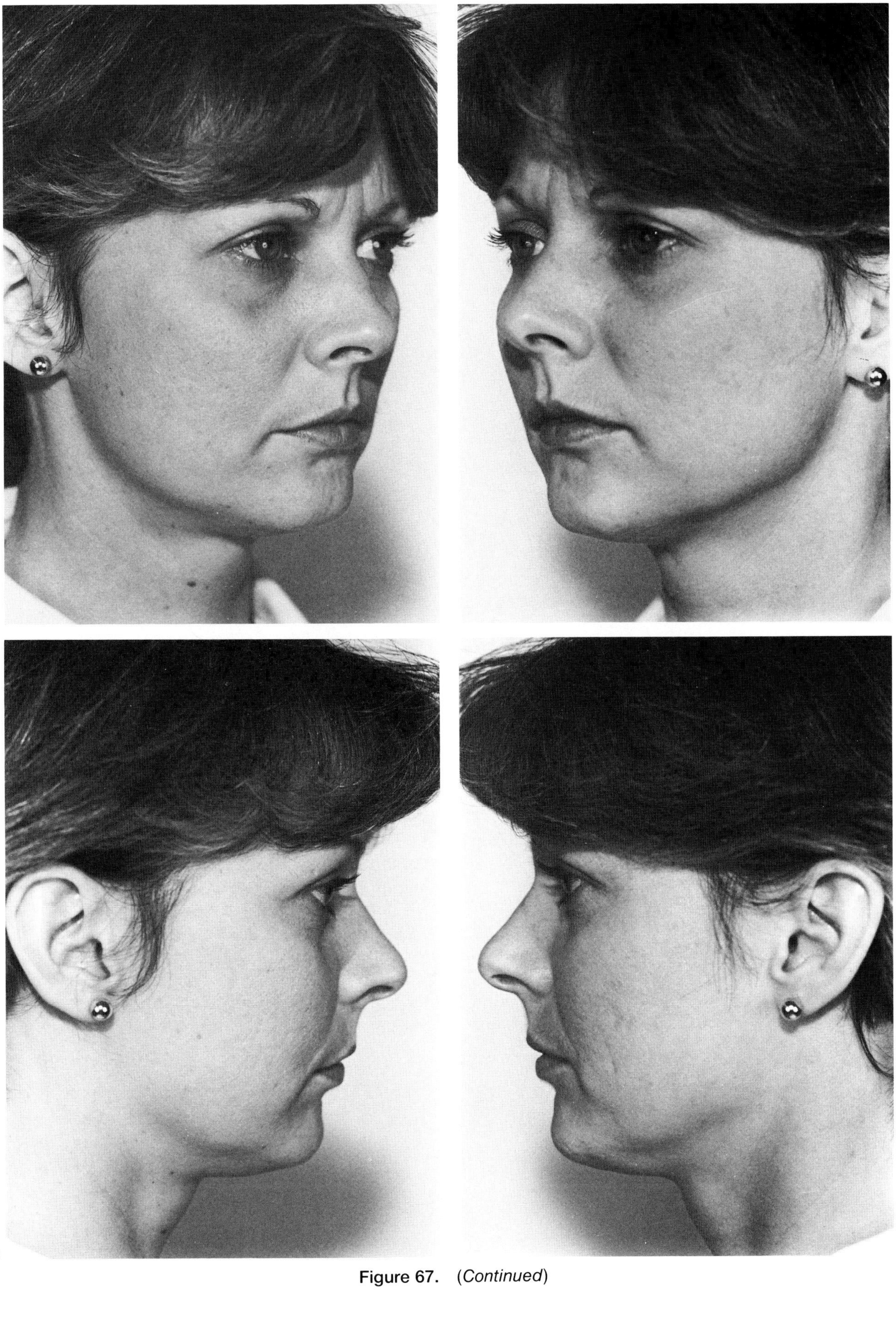

c d e f

Figure 67. (*Continued*)

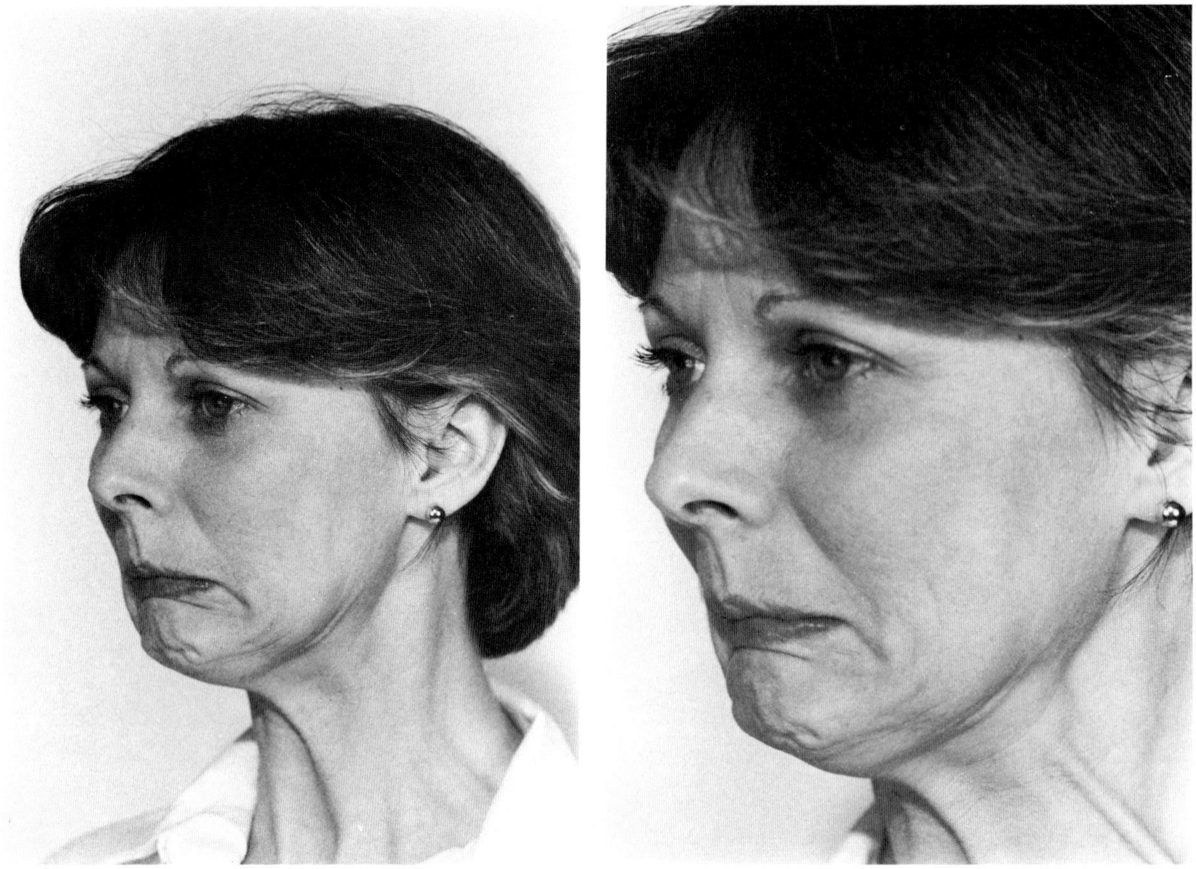

a b

Figure 68. a,b, An optional oblique view of forcible contraction of the mimetic musculature (particularly the platysma) may be useful in planning for appropriate lifting and tightening face-lift procedures.

FACIAL DEFORMITIES AND LESIONS

The exact nature of the abnormality will indicate the proper views to choose. In general, recommended views include:

1. Full face view (Fig. 69a)
2,3. Full face view—right or left lateral (Fig. 69b)
4,5. Full face view—right or left oblique (Fig. 69c)
6. Close-up view of abnormality (Fig. 69d)

If the abnormality is in the periorbital or perioral region, close-up views with eyes closed, lips pursed, or mouth open may be included for additional information. When in doubt, extra views should always be included, since after surgery the opportunity to record the preoperative condition is forever lost.

When recording close-up views of smaller lesions, it is usually helpful to include adjacent facial landmarks in the frame. For extreme close-ups, including a nondistracting, nonreflective centimeter rule is useful and informative to provide dimensions to the lesion (Fig. 70).

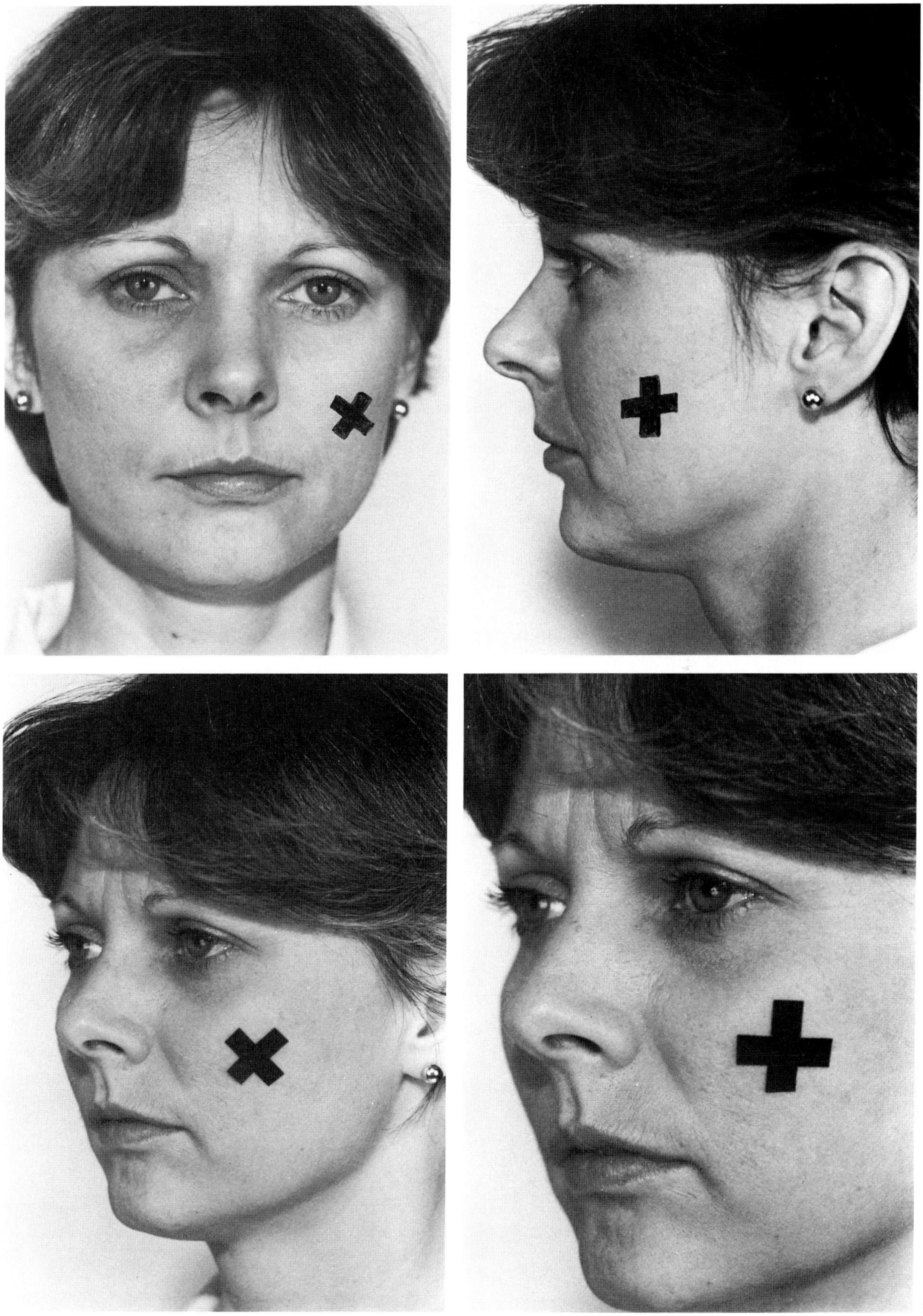

a b c d

Figure 69. a–d, Routine views recorded in patients with various facial conditions, lesions, or deformities. Additional views may be required, depending on the exact nature of the condition.

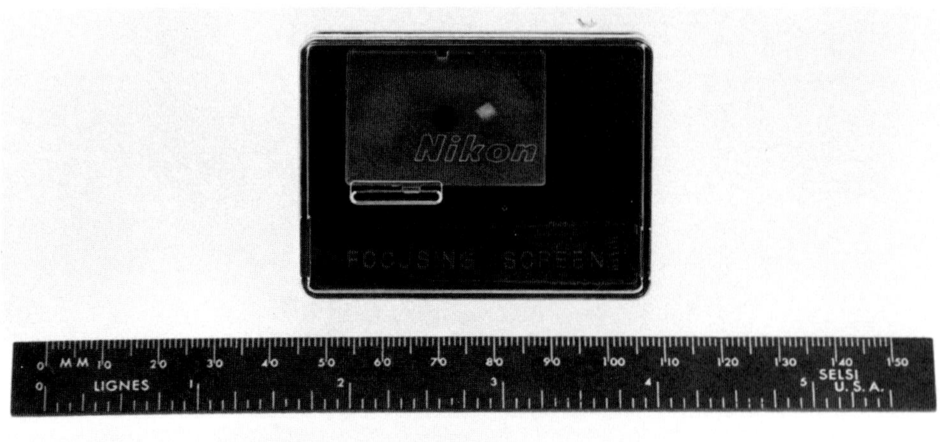

Figure 70. A nonreflecting centimeter rule positioned adjacent to the lesion or condition to be photographed is useful in judging proportion and dimension. It is always wise to include some adjacent identifying facial landmark in the recorded image to immediately orient the viewer.

SCARS

Undoubtedly, the most difficult condition to photograph properly and uniformly is the facial scar. Since scars are noticeable by virtue of the interplay of light and shadow effects surrounding them, lighting and exposure by the photographer will have a significant impact on the resultant photographic record. Moreover, recording the same scar in precisely the same manner before and after surgery is difficult at best. Intentional or inadvertent misrepresentation may easily occur by varying the lighting and exposure from sitting to sitting. Side lighting with slight underexposure may create significant shadow effects, overemphasizing the apparent magnitude of the scar; harsh frontal lighting with slight overexposure may spuriously improve the appearance of a surgical result. Striving for uniform lighting and exposure is difficult but highly desirable. Recording the aperture setting, light source angles, and distance from the lesion at the time of the initial photograph will provide a realistic guide for future accurate exposures.

Side or oblique lighting is clearly useful in documenting some facial scars that are less apparent in their magnitude to the patient when standard frontal lighting is used. No misrepresentation will occur if similar methods are used for the postoperative photographs.

Since facial animation may have a significant impact on the scar appearance, direction, and surgical planning for camouflage procedures, facial motion views are desirable. The following views for such scar documentation are recommended:

1. Full frontal view (Fig. 71a)
2. Close-up frontal view (Fig. 71b)
3. Lateral view (Fig. 71c)
4. Oblique view (Fig. 71d)

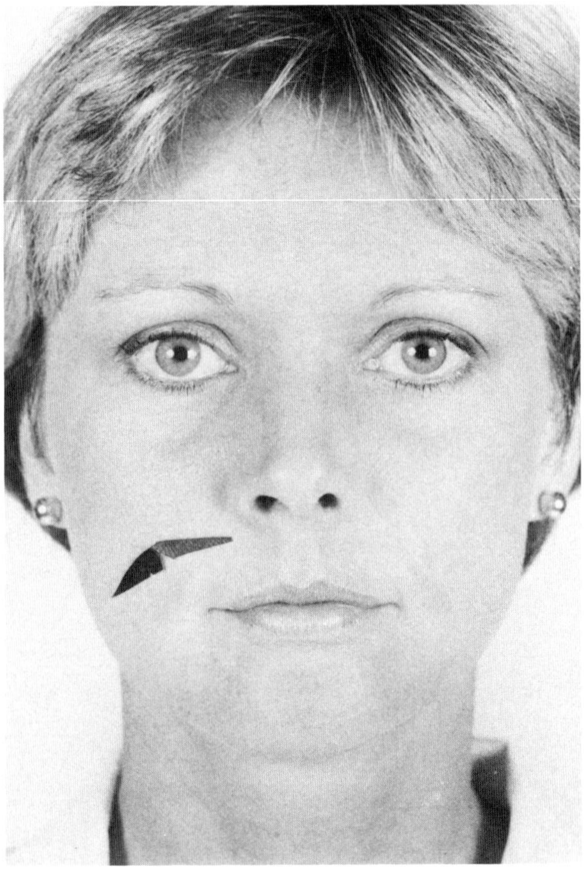

a

Figure 71. a–f, Recommended views for photographing facial scars. Of critical importance in achieving uniformity of exposure and positioning in scars is the strict adherence to the principles recommended for standard lighting, positioning, and framing. Tangential lighting to emphasize scar depressions or elevations may be dramatic, but often leads to unintentional photographic misrepresentation and is quite difficult to reproduce from sitting to sitting.

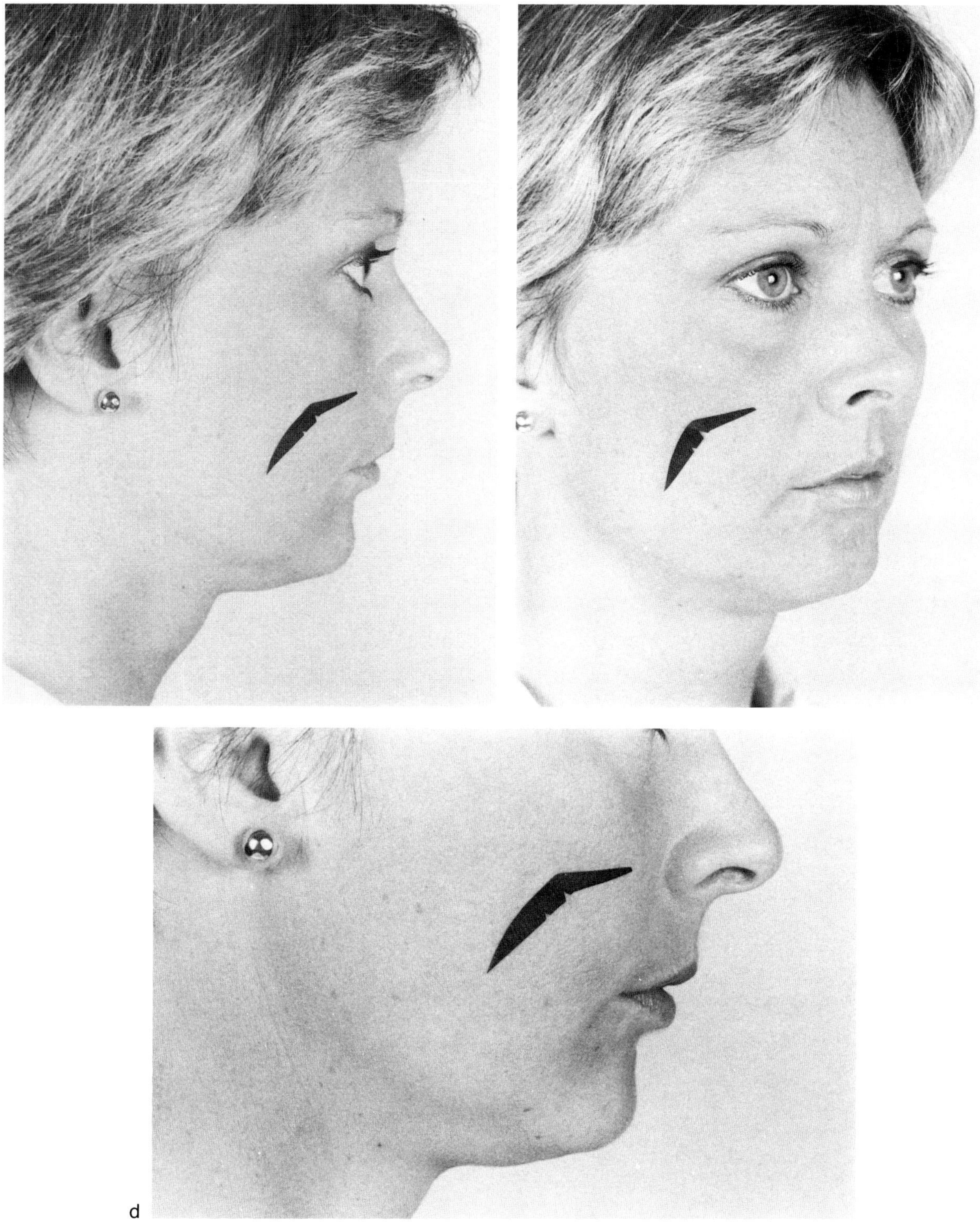

b c d

Figure 71. *(Continued)*

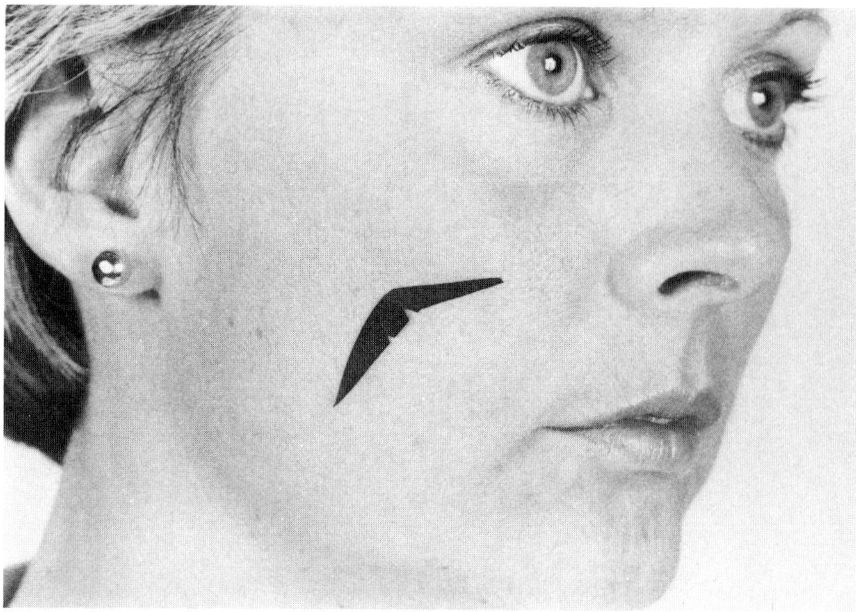

e

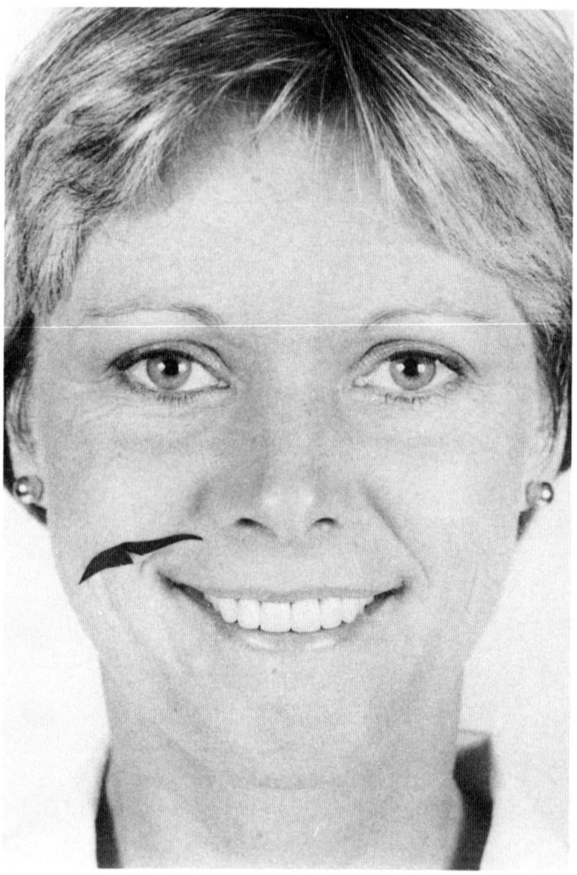

f

Figure 71. (*Continued*)

5. Close-up lateral and oblique views (if helpful) (Fig. 71d,e)
6. Appropriate views in animation (Fig. 71f)

When recording close-up views, the principle of including recognizable landmarks in the area surrounding the scar is helpful.

OTOPLASTY AND EAR DEFORMITIES

Documenting ear abnormalities requires extra attention to detail. Hair must not obscure proper appreciation of the ear anatomy from either the front or posterior view. Colored elastic headbands, barrettes, and hair clips arranged unobtrusively will control long hair nicely. The same technique and arrangement should be utilized postoperatively to avoid distracting clutter and nonuniformity.

Useful in documenting the ear anatomy are seven views:

1. Frontal face view (Fig. 72a)
2. Posterior head view (Fig. 72b)
3,4. Right and left lateral close-up views (Fig. 72c,d)
5,6. Right and left oblique close-up views (Fig. 72e,f)
7. Submental vertex (Fig. 72g)

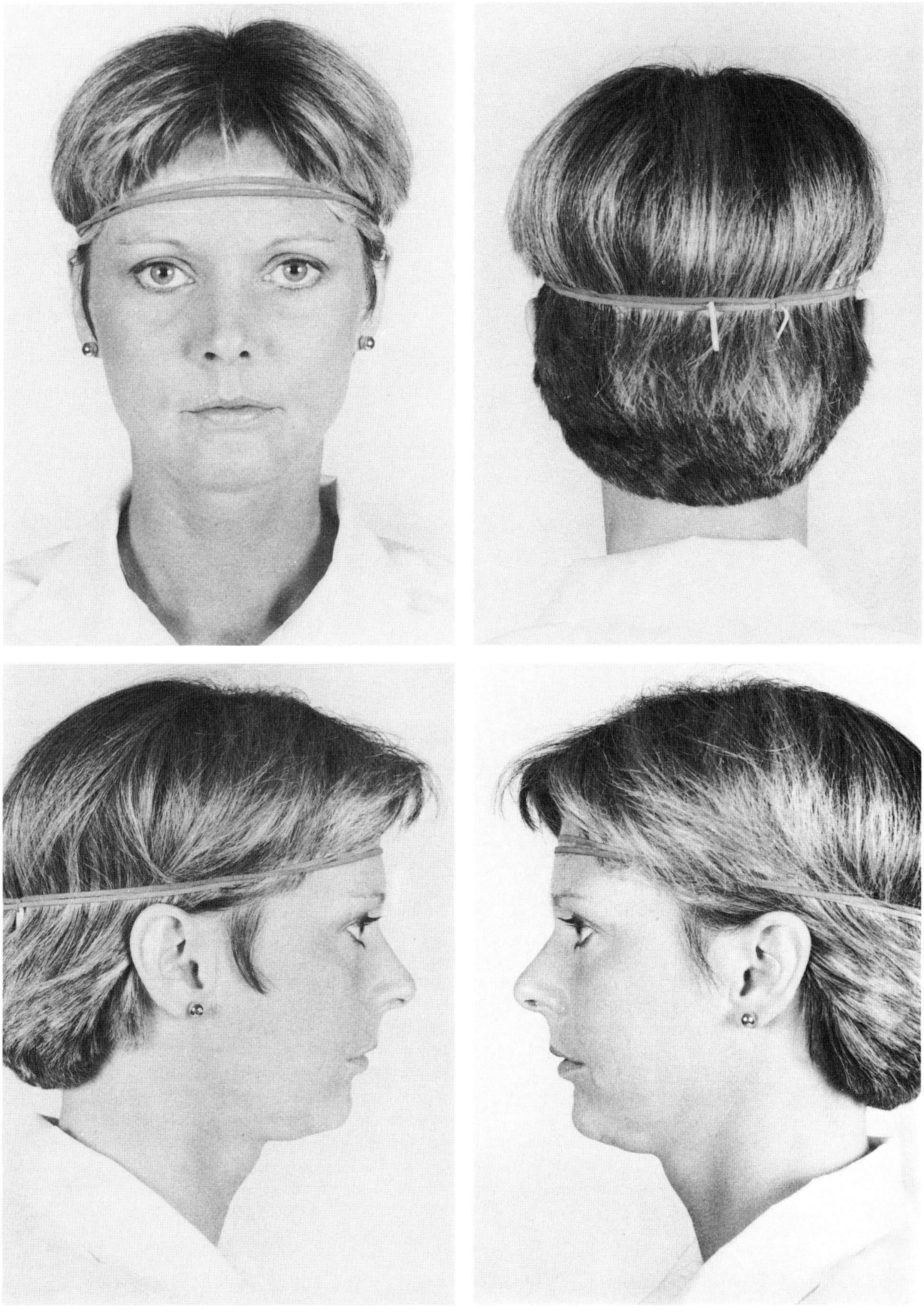

a b c d

Figure 72. **a–g,** Routine views recommended for the patient undergoing otoplasty or correction of auricular deformities. Control of the hair is critical in these views, and symmetry of positioning absolutely essential to avoid unintentional photographic misrepresentation.

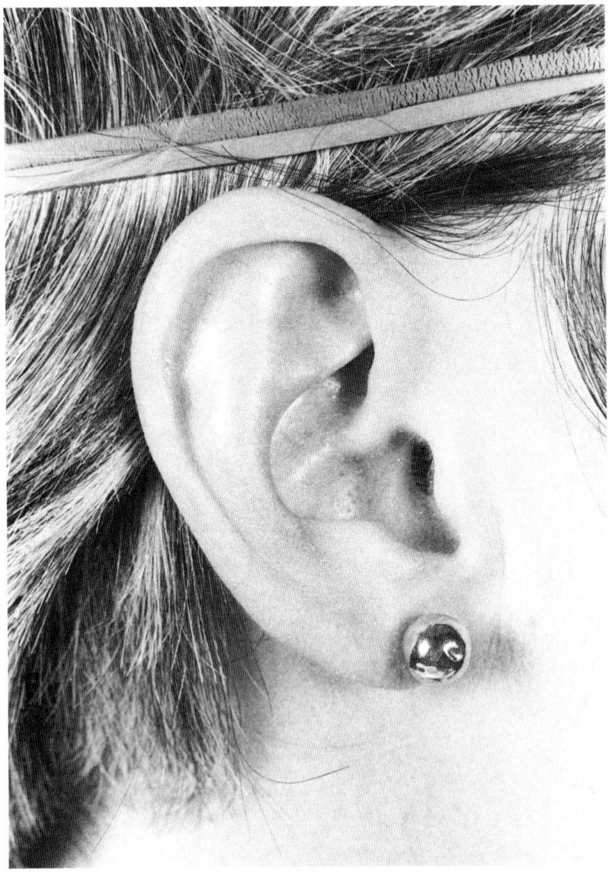

e

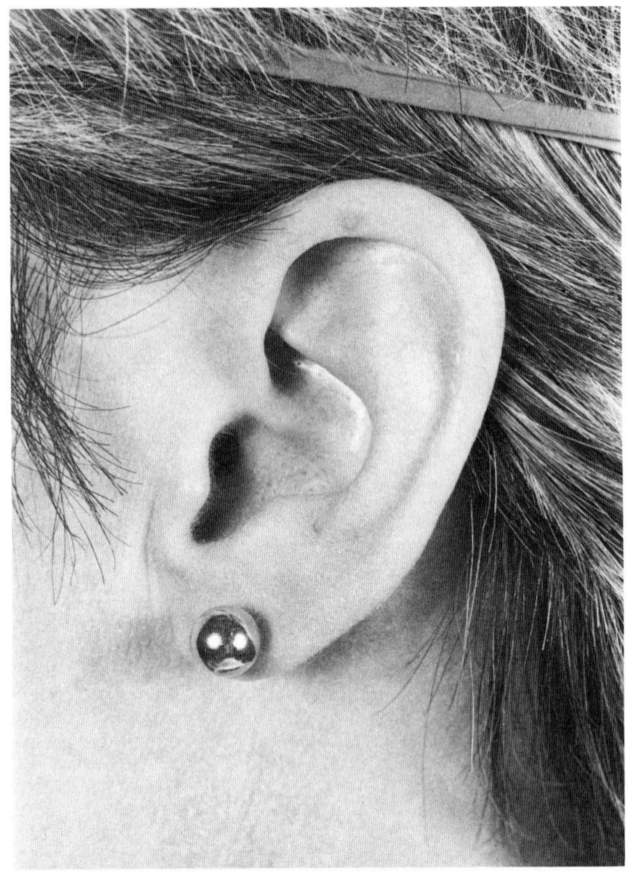

f

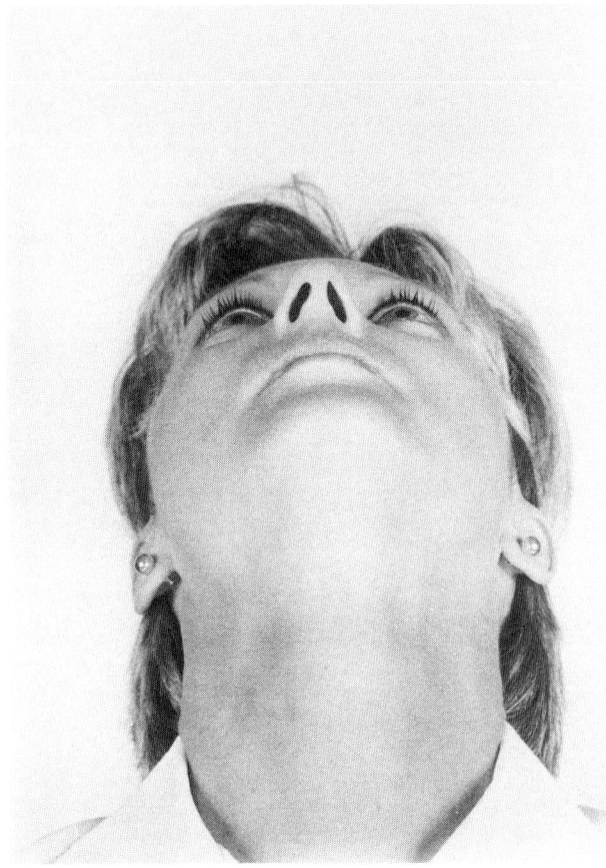

g

Figure 72. (*Continued*)

Close attention must be paid to the midsagittal line on frontal and posterior views to reflect the ear-head position accurately without distortion. Even slight head rotation from the midsagittal line on a frontal view will influence the apparent anterior or posterior position of the auricle.

MENTOPLASTY AND SUBMENTOPLASTY

Useful views, which must include the neck, are:

1. Full frontal view (Fig. 73a)
2. Close-up lateral view (Fig. 73b)
3. Right and left lateral views (Fig. 73c,d)

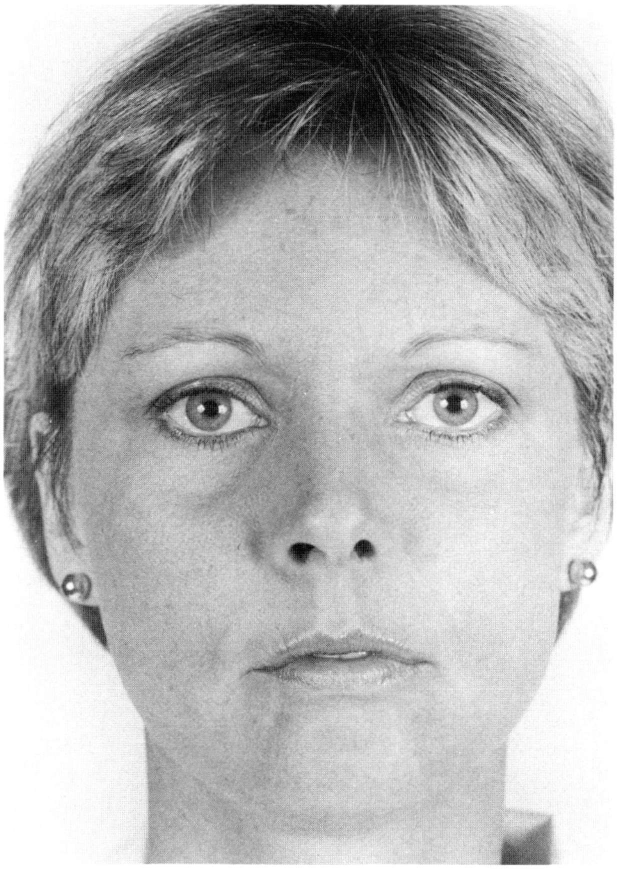

a

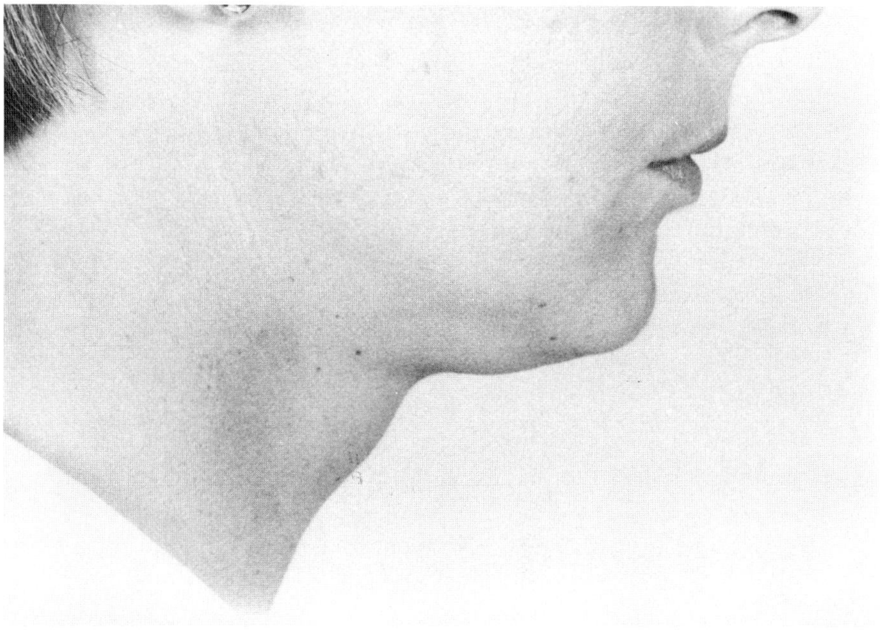

b

Figure 73. a–d, Recommended views for mentoplasty and submentoplasty procedures. An optional view might include one demonstrating, with a forced contortional grimace, the activity and dynamic anatomy of the submental platysma.

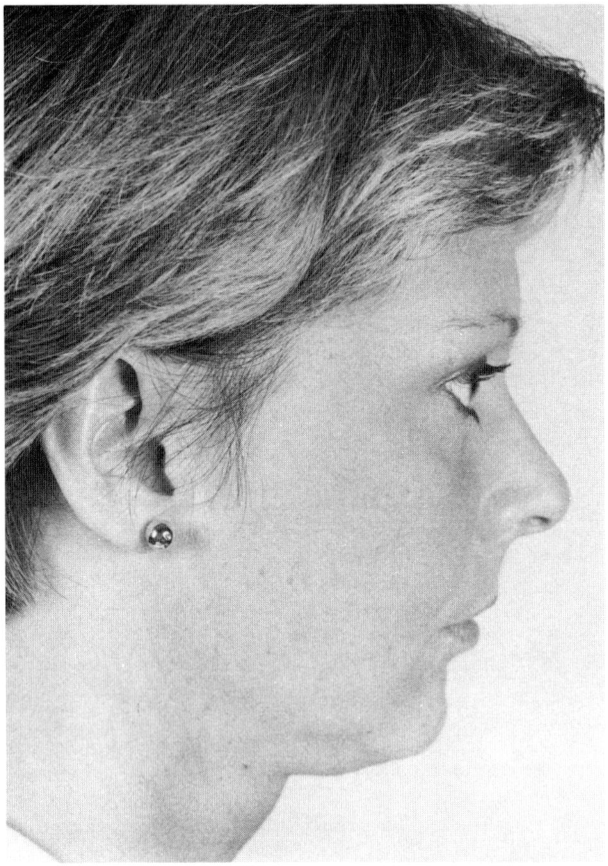

c

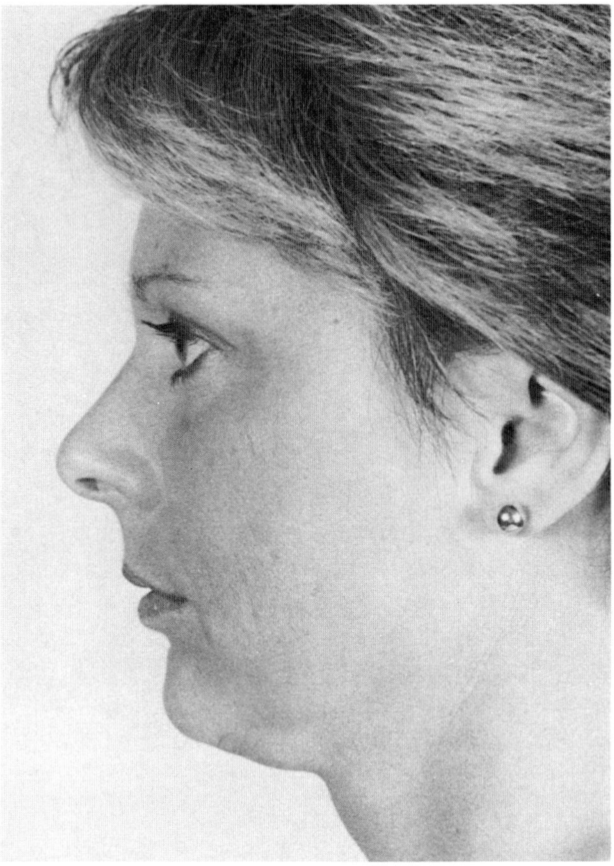

d

Figure 73. (*Continued*)

SCALP (HAIR TRANSPLANT)

Pre- and postoperative photographs of hair transplantation procedures are often inaccurately recorded. This regrettable discrepancy may be overcome by uniformly obtaining the following recommended views:

1. Full face view (Fig. 74a)
2. Full head view—posterior (Fig. 74b)
3. Head down with hair swept away from involved area (Fig. 74c)
4. Head down with hair combed to camouflage defect (Fig. 74d)

In specific lesions or conditions involving smaller areas of the scalp, additional close-up views are recommended.

MALPOSITION AVOIDANCE

Positioning errors are particularly common in facial photography and may add to significant nonuniformity and misrepresentation (Fig. 75a-l). Patients must be constantly reminded to sit erect (avoiding leaning forward or backward), and look straight ahead, preferably at a premarked image on the wall. The constant tendency is to gaze upward, and in so doing, lift the chin and neck upward. The Frankfort horizontal line must be rigidly imposed to avoid this tendency (Fig. 75m).

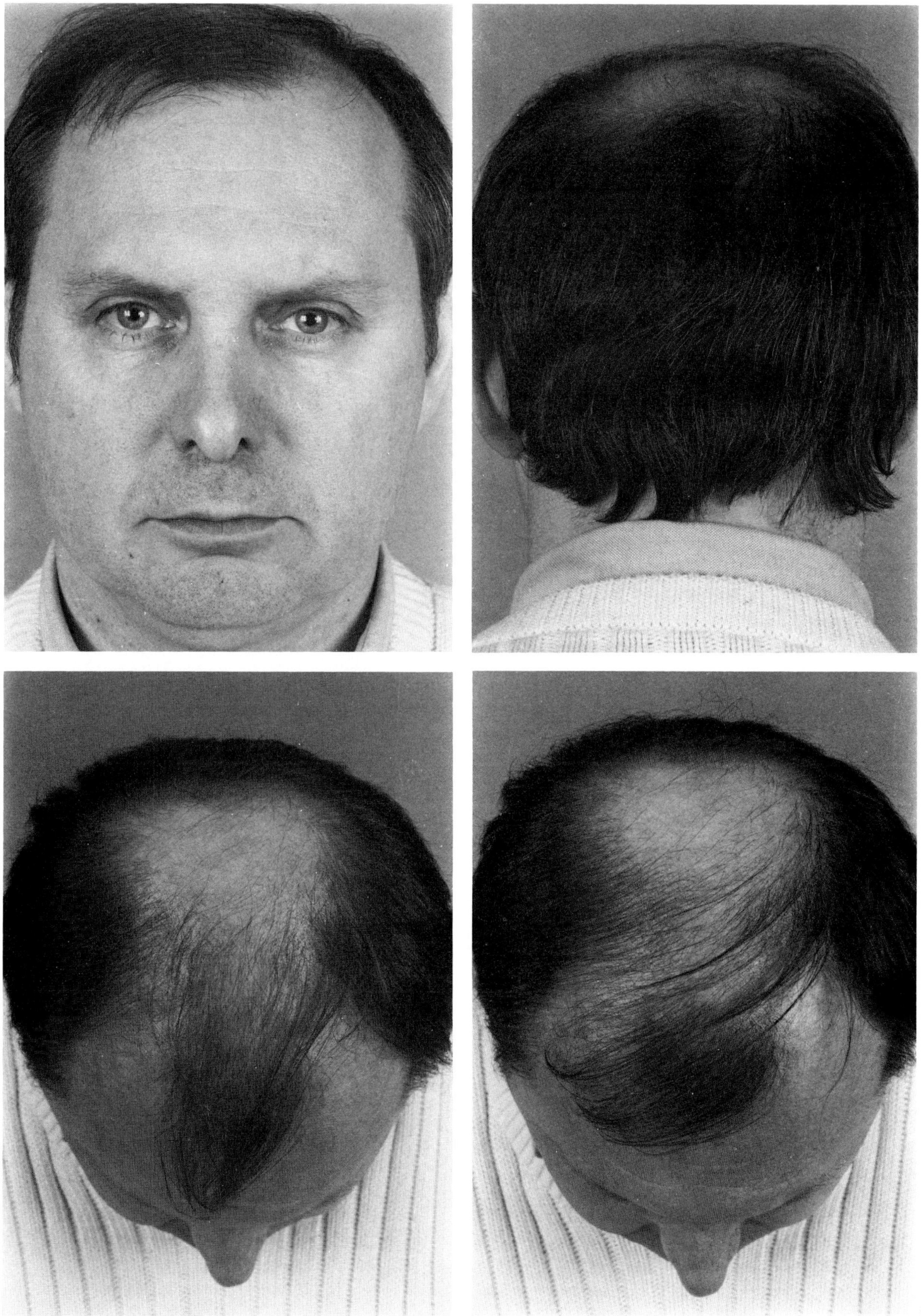

a b c d

Figure 74. **a–d,** Recommended views for patients undergoing hair transplantation.

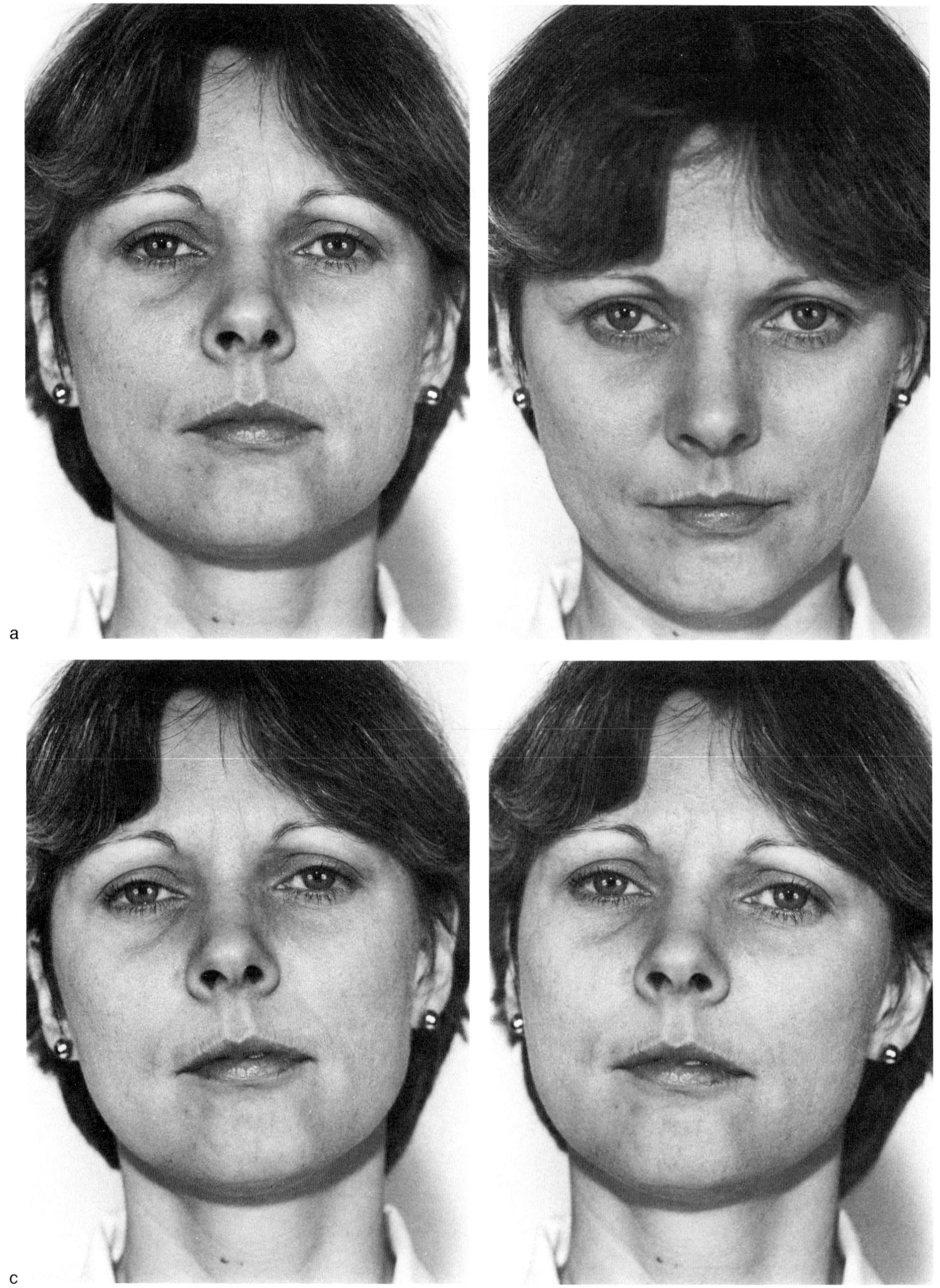

Figure 75. Positional errors abound in facial photography. **a,** The subject's head is tilted backward, giving the appearance of a shorter nasal length. **b,** Subject's head is tilted downward, spuriously elongating the nose. **c,** Head is tilted to right. **d,** Head is tilted to left.

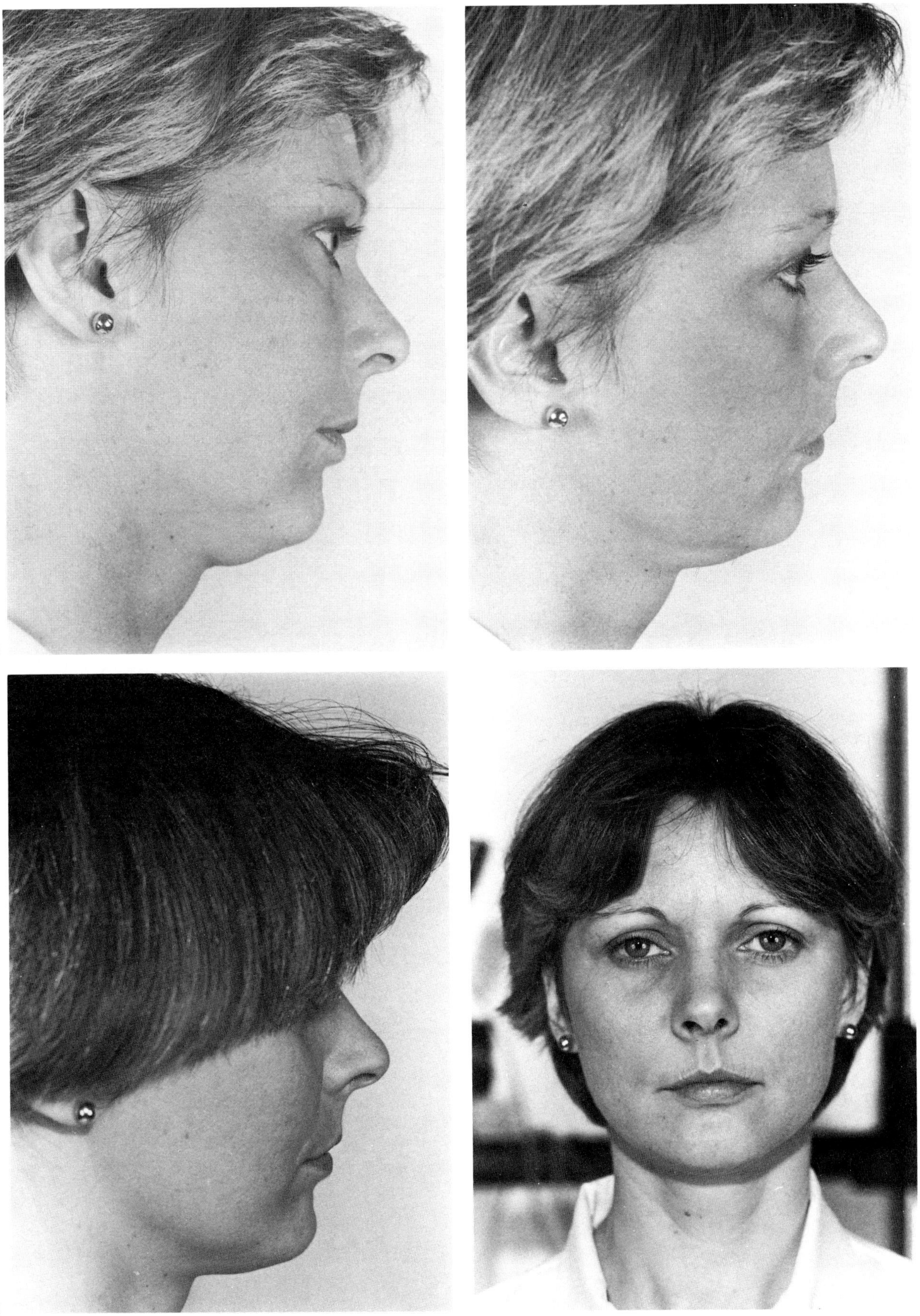

Figure 75. (*Continued*) **e,** Head is tilted away from the camera on the lateral view, spuriously changing the nasal profile and alar-columellar relationship. **f,** Head is tilted toward camera on lateral view, with similar spurious relationship changes. **g,** Major details of face and nose are obscured by uncontrolled hair. **h,** Cluttered, distracting, nonuniform background.

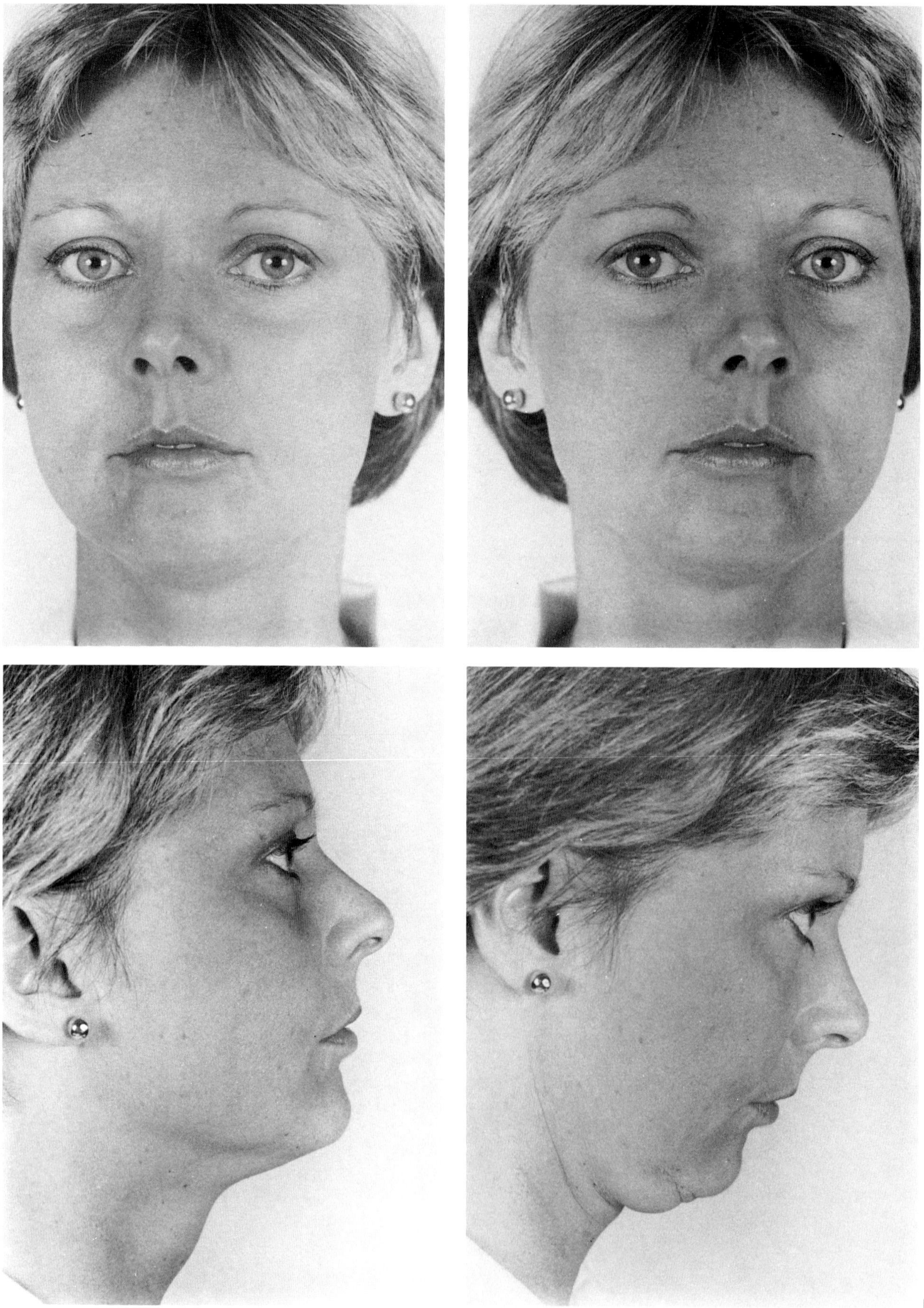

i j k l

Figure 75. (*Continued*) **i,** Head is rotated to right, with more auricle visible on one side than the other. **j,** Head is rotated to left, again revealing more auricle unilaterally and suggesting a slight nasal twist where none exists. **k,** Head is tilted upward on lateral view (probably the single most common error made in patient positioning), due to failure to observe the Frankfort horizontal line in aligning the patient's head. The majority of patients tend to angle the head upward when sitting for lateral photographs and must be constantly reminded to look straight ahead. **l,** Head tilted downward, below plane of Frankfort line.

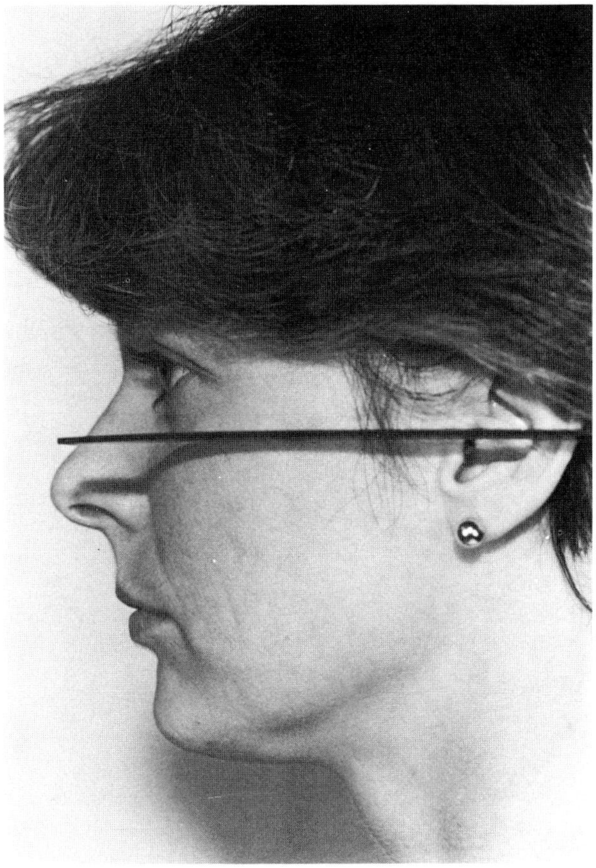

m

Figure 75. *(Continued)* **m,** Frankfort horizontal line.

OPERATING ROOM PHOTOGRAPHY

Every surgical photograph should, on its own, tell a story (Fig. 76a). The image that emphasizes a specific and, ideally, complete thought or principle is a powerful teaching tool (Fig. 76b).

A single photograph can reveal in a most vivid fashion and in "living color" the surgeon's operative plan, his predetermined alternative possibilities, and even the illusion of motion (Fig. 77a-c) (the latter capability is particularly enhanced if sequential photographs are recorded with precisely uniform framing of the component steps of an operation). Arrows drawn on the skin (they should be delicate and not overwhelm the principal surgical problem) add life and motion to an operative event, visually introducing the events to follow (Fig. 78). Areas to be excised or undermined may be so indicated by using a light-marking pen and crosshatching (Fig. 79). Planned incisions may be indicated by lightly drawn, incomplete lines (Fig. 80); the addition of a different colored sterile marking pen can be even more dramatic if the effect is not overdone (Fig. 81).

Scrupulously following a few simple but critical rules will enhance any operating room photograph. Bleeding—even minimal oozing—must be controlled, and bloody towels and sponges (Fig. 82a) removed from the framed field and replaced with fresh towels of the same color and texture (Fig. 82b). Shades of blue or green are best and gray is not objectionable, but white towels and sponges create a distracting glare by reflecting light and are thus poor choices (Fig. 83). The drape framing should include a familiar orienting landmark (Fig. 84a,b), such as an eyebrow, an ear, an identifiable component of the nose, for instant and graphic reference sources to aid understanding by potential viewers. If landmarks are indistinct (e.g., in neck surgery), identifying skeletal structures (hyoid, thyroid cartilage, midsternal notch) can be marked for orientation (Fig. 85a-b).

Towel clips and shiny surgical instruments should be kept out of the field when possible to eliminate glare and distraction (Fig. 86a). If available, ebonized or matte dull finish instruments (Richards Medical Company) are photographically superior

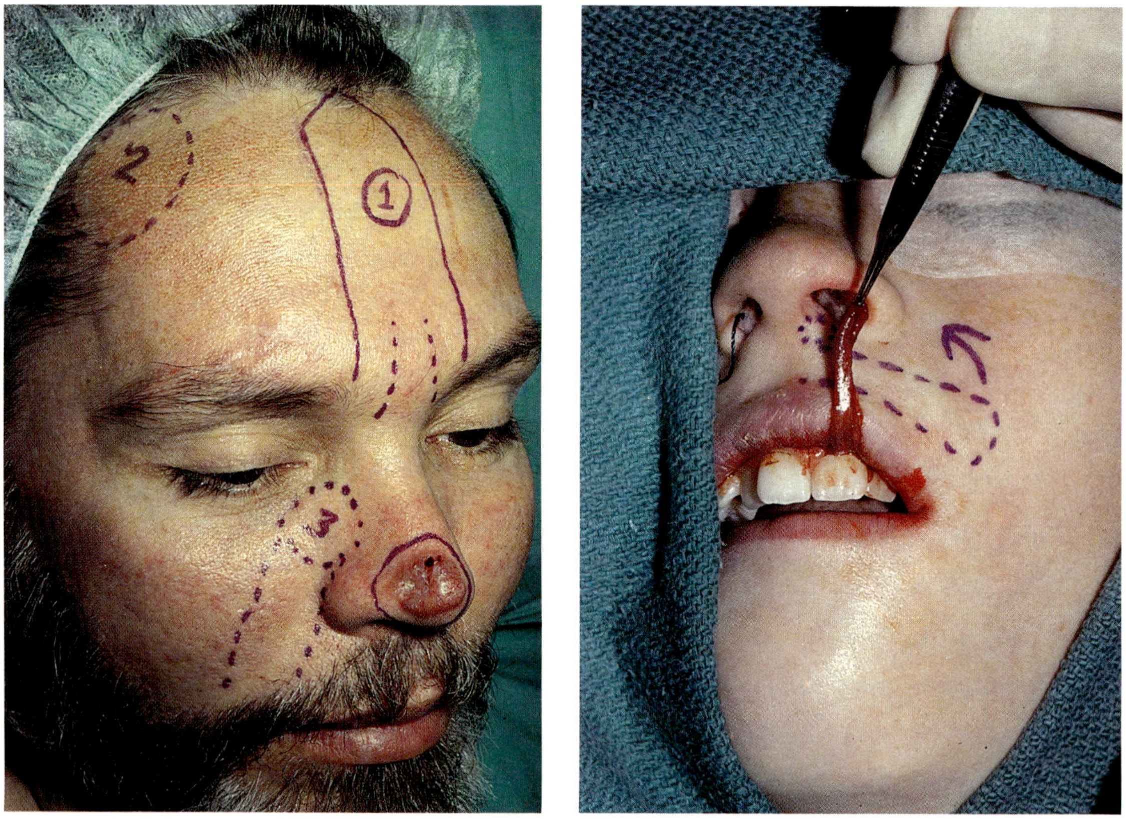

a b

Figure 76. a,b, Ideal operating room photographs should contain teaching messages or principles that are vivid and self-evident to even the unsophisticated viewer. Introducing a certain amount of "thought control" will enhance the value of photographic communication and may eliminate the need for prolonged explanations or additional photographs to complete a thought.

(Fig. 86b). If sponges are necessary to include for some reason (e.g., in surgical television), light blue tinted 4 × 4 sponges serve best. In general, gloved fingers are best eliminated from the field, but when this is not possible, brown gloves are preferred to standard white surgical gloves, creating less distraction and glare.

Further information can be added to surgical photographs by placing a graphic but unobtrusive centimeter rule at the periphery of the field (Fig. 87). It, too, should be nonreflective, clearly readable, and preferably not include an advertisement for the company who manufactures it. If vessels or nerves are being photographed, some method to separate them visually from the background tissues is helpful (Fig. 88). Passing a small instrument, Q-tip, tongue blade, large suture, or colored paper between the structure and its background tissues will enhance its visibility and therefore improve recognition and understanding.

Operative photographs are usually best taken from the viewpoint and orientation of the operating surgeon (Fig. 89a-d). Since in teaching, most photographs will be viewed predominantly by surgeons, departures from normal orientation from the surgeon's viewpoint may be more than momentarily confusing, diminishing their educational impact.

Finally, it is recommended that the best operating room photographic results are usually obtained when a generous number of bracketed views are taken at the operating table. Now is not the time to be stingy with film. Inevitably, some shots will be superior to others, and it is only by careful planning combined with exposure bracketing that consistently appealing and superior photographs are obtained. Only one chance exists to record such operative events; that opportunity is instantly and forever lost as the operation proceeds.

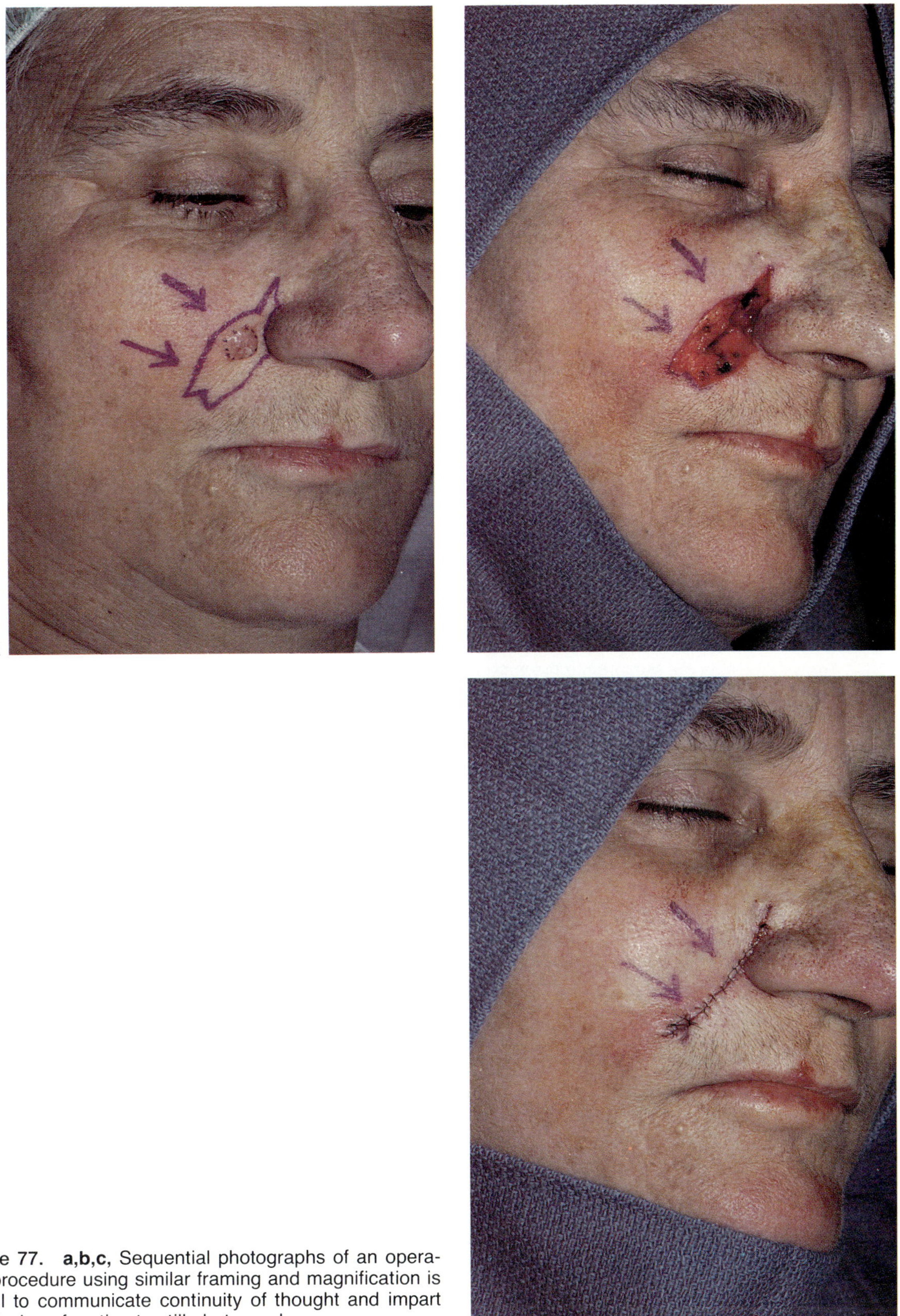

Figure 77. **a,b,c,** Sequential photographs of an operative procedure using similar framing and magnification is useful to communicate continuity of thought and impart the illusion of motion to still photographs.

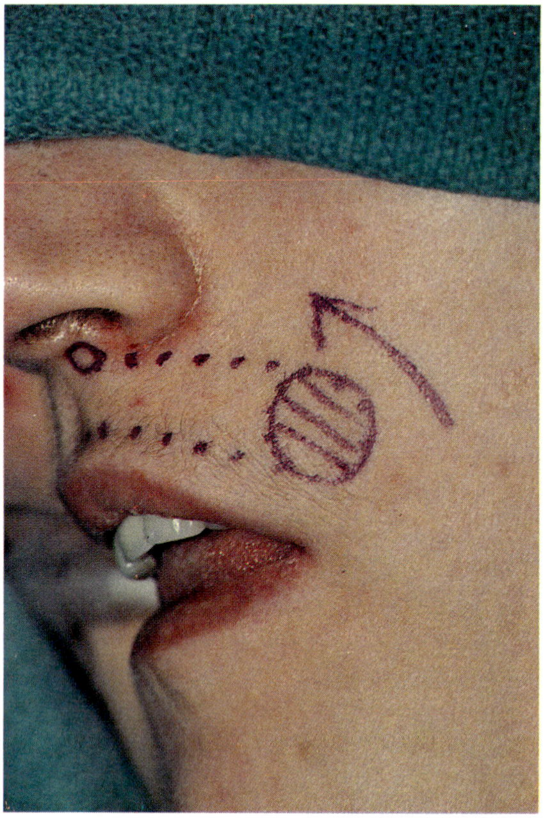

Figure 78. Arrows drawn on the skin prior to the incision impart a fluidity to the intended procedure, providing a strong clue to the dynamics of the operation. The illusion of motion is created.

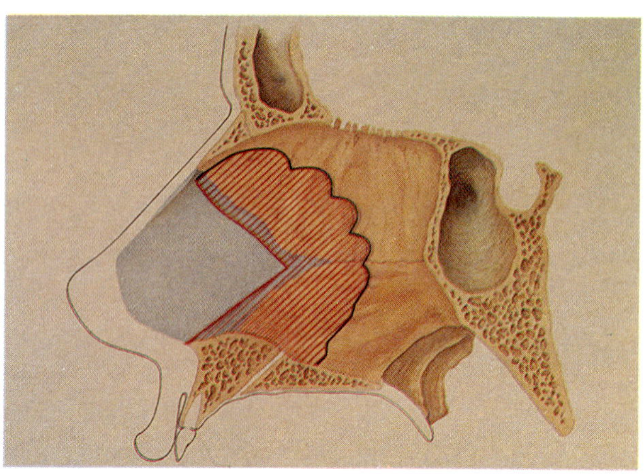

Figure 79. Crosshatching clearly indicates the areas to be excised or removed.

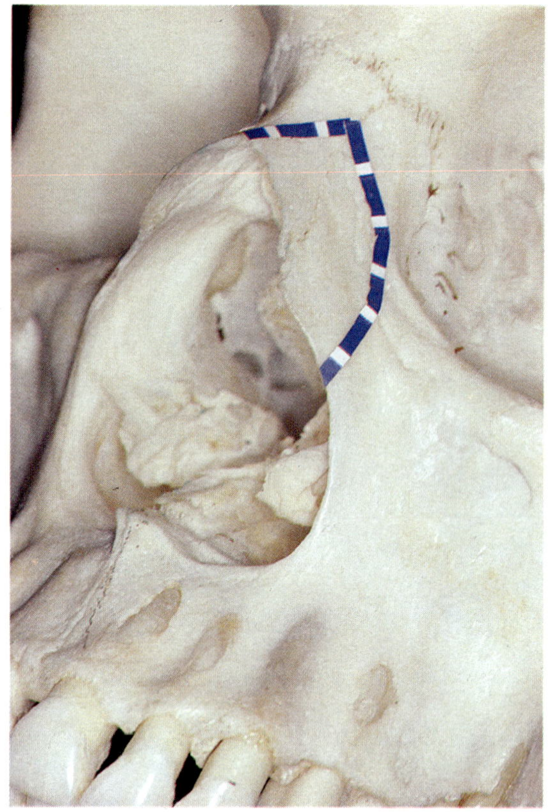

Figure 80. Dotted or incomplete lines have universal recognition as the lines of intended incisions.

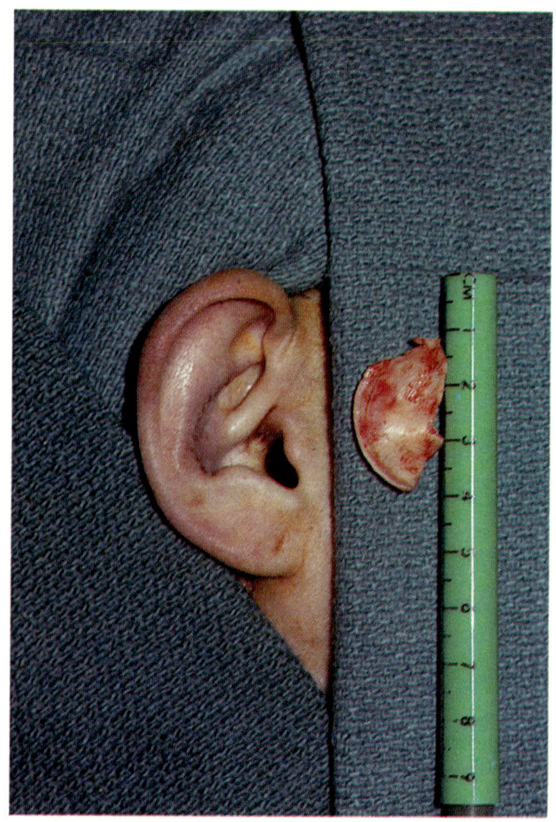

Figure 81. Introducing color into the field to be operated on adds additional information and drama to the operative photograph.

a 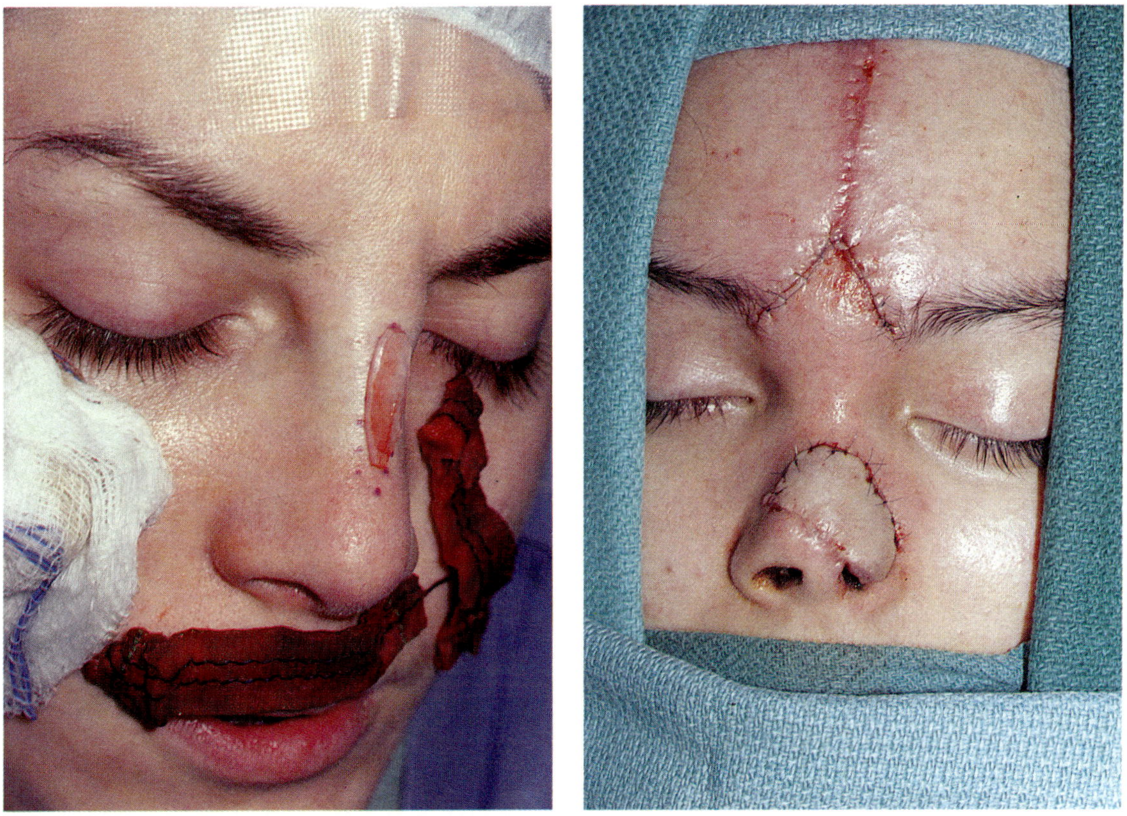 b

Figure 82. a,b, Any operative field should be free of blood and extraneous instruments and sponges in order to record the most meaningful, clear image. Fresh towels of identical color should be properly draped and all blood, which absorbs light, removed.

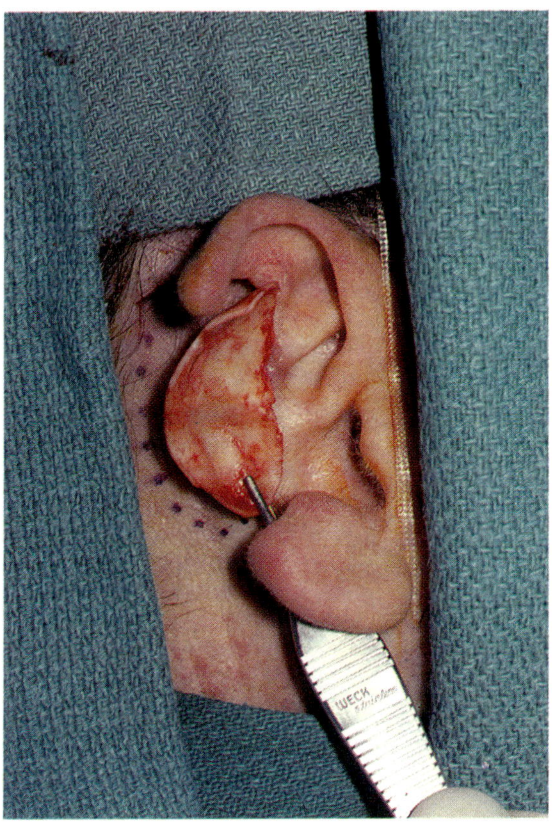

Figure 83. In general, white towels may create glare and are best replaced with towels of more neutral shades (green, blue, or gray)

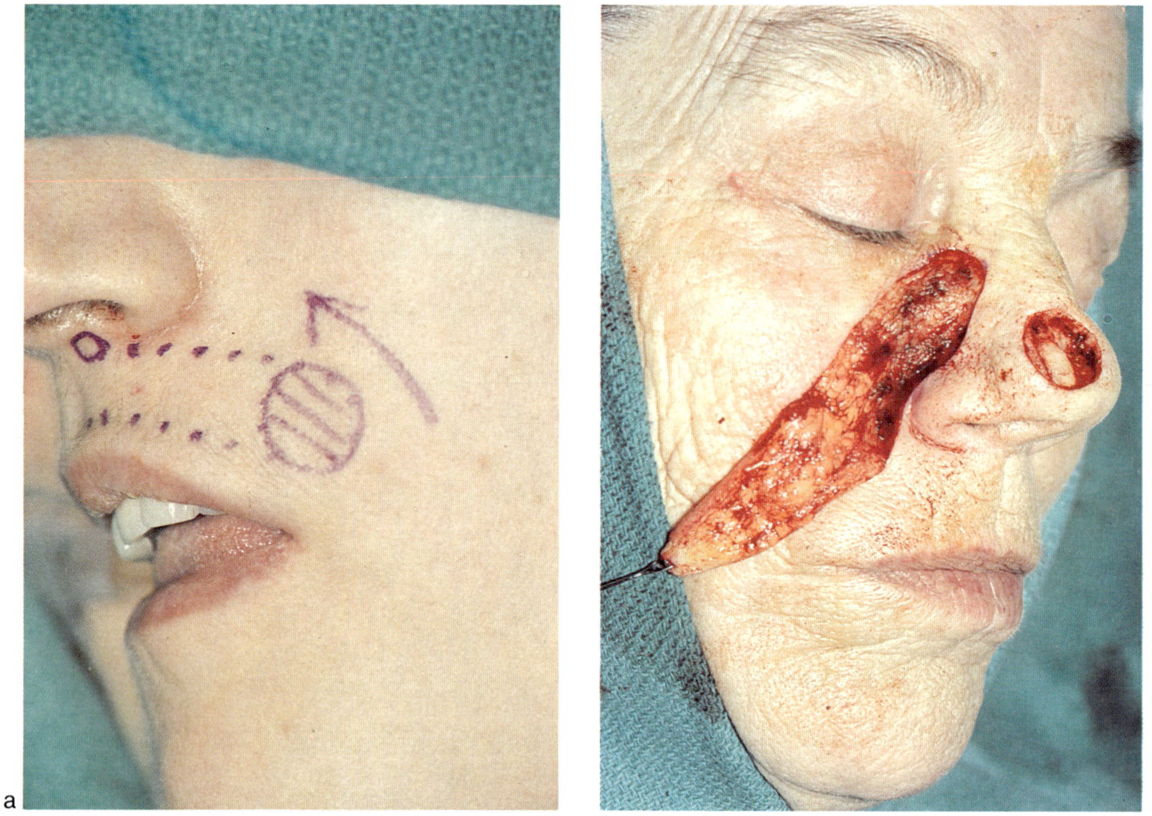

Figure 84. **a,b,** In the face, the inclusion of orienting adjacent landmarks in the field to be draped and photographed is helpful.

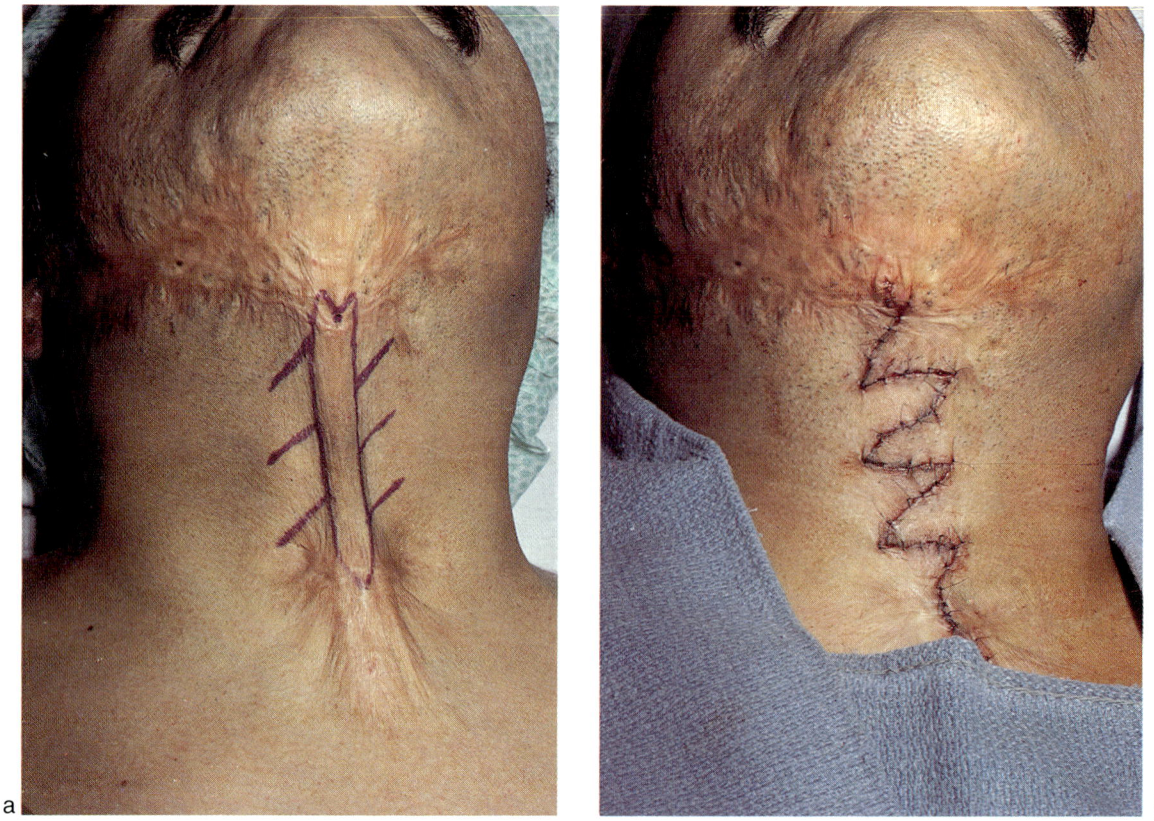

Figure 85. **a,b,** In the neck, landmarks such as the hyoid and thyroid cartilages or the suprasternal notch will help instantly to orient the viewer.

a 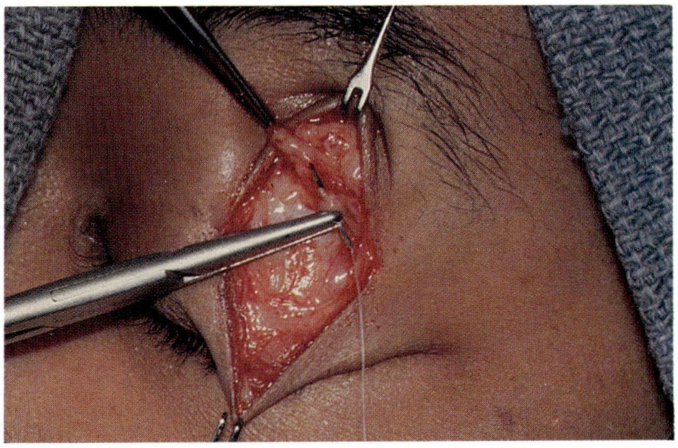 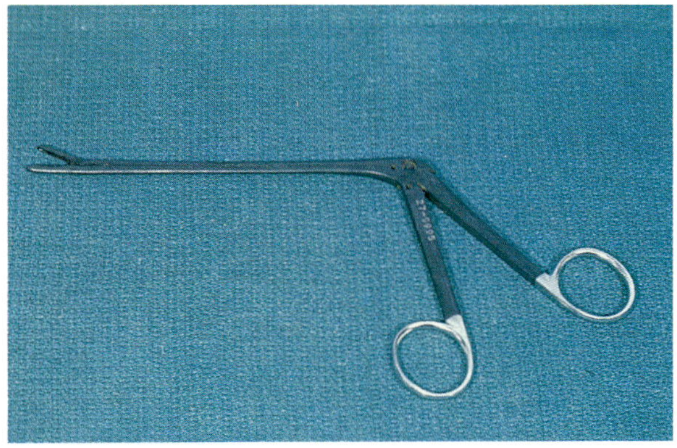 b

Figure 86. **a,** Shiny instruments in the operating field often reflect light and produce unwanted glare. **b,** Ebonized instruments eliminate this undesirable characteristic.

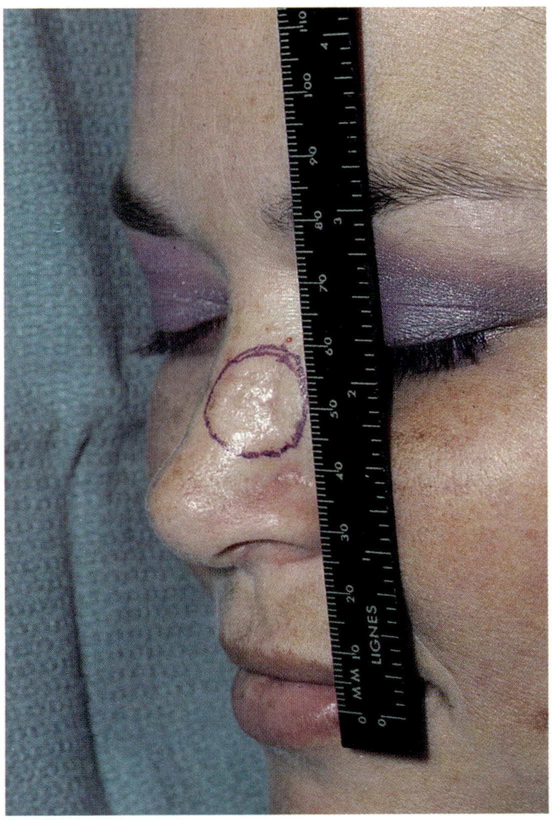

Figure 87. A nonreflective centimeter rule placed adjacent to the central theme of the photograph, or in the periphery of the frame, is useful to orient the viewer quickly to linear dimensions.

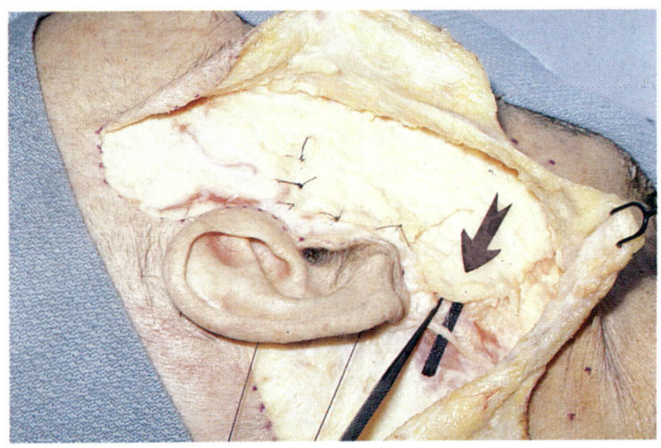

Figure 88. Since vessels or nerves often become visually lost in the background of a dissected operative field, placing some object of contrasting color or shape between the anatomic feature of interest and the background will serve to isolate and highlight it.

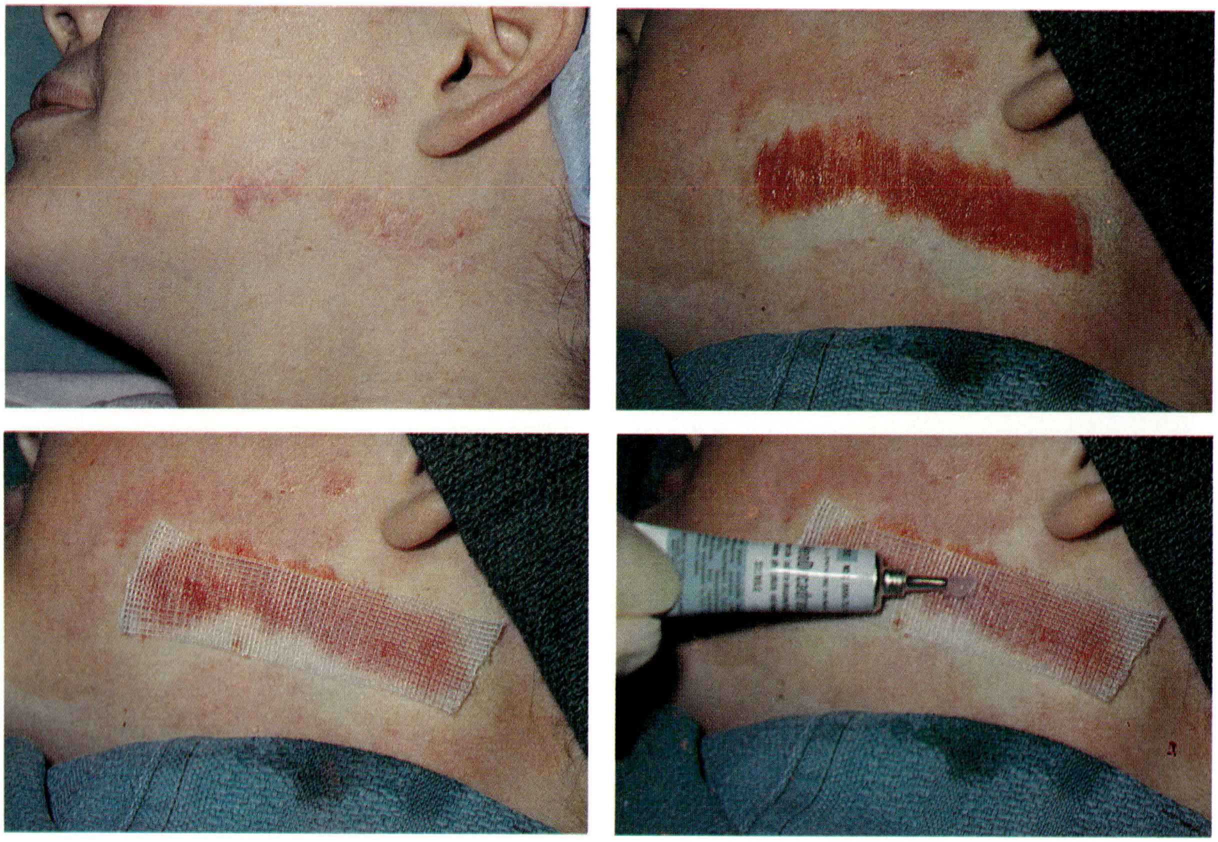

a b c d

Figure 89. **a,b,c,d,** Operative photographs, especially when taken in sequence to demonstrate the steps of an operative procedure, are best taken uniformly from the usual viewpoint and orientation of the operating surgeon.

5 The Creative Process

THE PHOTOESSAY

All presentations incorporating visual aids supplemented by a vocal presentation (or vice versa) are in reality photoessays. Every presentation (regardless of the subject or length of the presentation) makes a statement about the speaker. A carelessly prepared and executed scientific presentation leaves a lingering doubt in the minds of the audience about that physician's overall competence. Even worse, the ordeal may represent an affront to an audience eager to learn. The well-prepared, informative, and entertaining speaker is universally perceived as organized and expert in his medical capabilities as a whole. Exceptions to these truisms, of course, exist, but they are uncommon. Good speakers strive for an economy of words and phrases, relying on vivid visual aids to clarify and augment the spoken word. Striking individual visual images often become more firmly fixed in the learner's mind than several paragraphs of scientific rhetoric (Figs. 90,91). In contemporary continuing education, the presentor commonly is required to deliver his opinions and results in 10- to 15-minute segments, with little time to qualify, augment, clarify, or justify his thinking.

Memorable visual aids serve to solidify concepts of vital importance (Figs. 92,93). Slides containing even one or a few key words and concepts can be extremely effective (Figs. 94,95). This becomes even more critical when speaking to a lay audience, who have a limited frame of reference to the subject than do medical specialists.

Even the occasional speaker needs to develop a style of excellence in creating and delivering the photoessay. It is important that the visual aids never overwhelm or distract from a principal message; they should augment and catalyze the communication process. Certain principles of visual presentation are worthy of emphasis and will be explored here.

More often than not, a scientific meeting presentation is delivered as a distillate of a larger, detailed manuscript. The latter work, when published, will contain details and elaborations of the scientific project, experiment, or technique upon which the author wishes to report. Less stringent limitations are imposed for journal publishing than for the finite spoken presentation.

The effective speaker must prepare two manuscripts: one for eventual publication and another, attenuated and concentrated, for verbal and visual presentation. To fit concisely within the allotted time frame, the presented paper must be lean and spare, with an economy of words and phrases. This requirement is best met by the liberal but carefully select use of effective visual aids—most commonly, the 35 mm color transparency. With fewer words and more visual elements, communication of ideas is most easily understood and fixed in the listener's and viewer's mind.

A spoken presentation should highlight, in capsule form, the main features of the entire manuscript, wasting no phrase or visual opportunity. An economy of words, phrases, and details is of utmost importance. It should be accurately timed and retimed in advance by reading it aloud at a comfortable speaking rate, allowing time to add explanations, if required, about the simultaneously shown visual aids. If the allotted time for the presentation is 15 minutes, the manuscript should fit easily into a 14-minute time frame, allowing for introductory comments of the chairman, the speaker's walk to the podium, and any possible delay occasioned by audio or projection difficulties.

A few sacred guidelines to presentation preparation are worthy of emphasis. The opening sentence is of critical importance, as its sole purpose is to capture the audience's attention instantly. The traditionally historical opening sentence ("Jacques Joseph is considered the father of rhinoplasty") may interest a few but will seldom capture the attention generated by a startling, negative, or contrasting statement. The startling statement, "The number of master rhinoplasty surgeons in the world may be counted on two hands," may or may not be absolutely accurate, but will surely provoke interest. The contrast statement, "Many surgeons may perform rhinoplasty, but few ever master the procedure," is difficult to refute. Quotations can stimu-

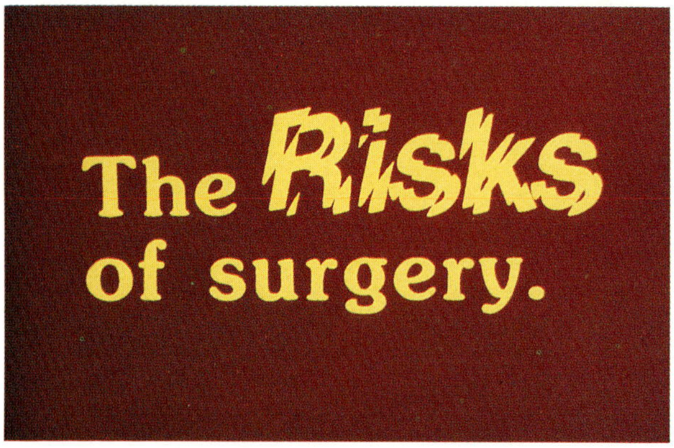

Figure 90. One striking visual presentation may be more meaningful than paragraphs of dialogue or rhetoric in medical communication.

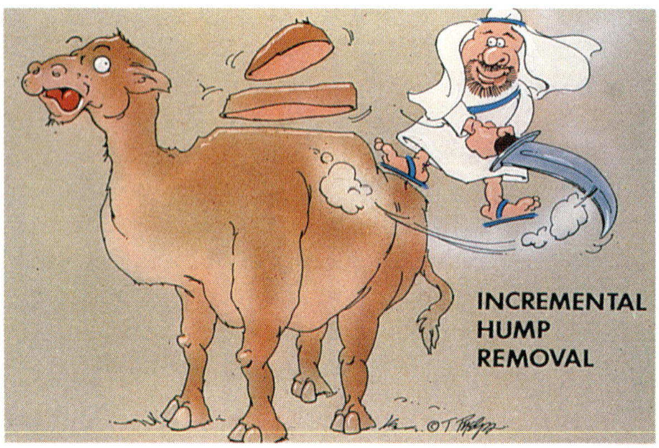

Figure 91. An effective striking visual image.

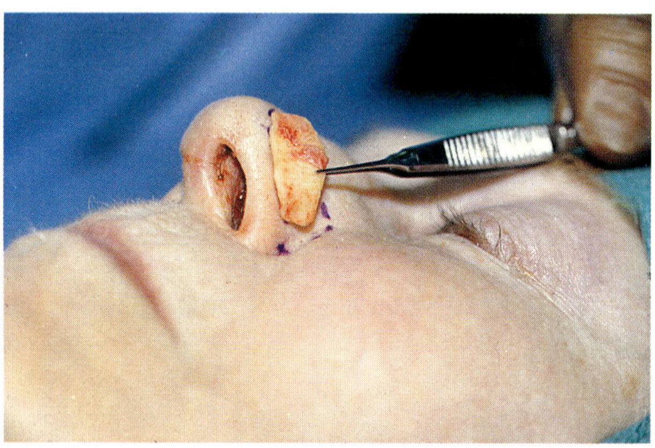

Figure 92. Visual material that communicates a thought clearly.

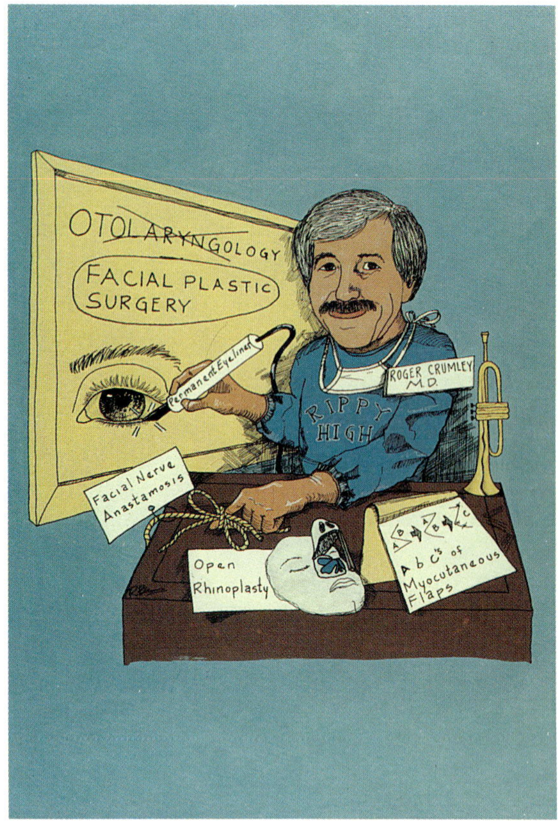

Figure 93. Attention-getting visual aid, designed to attract and hold audience interest.

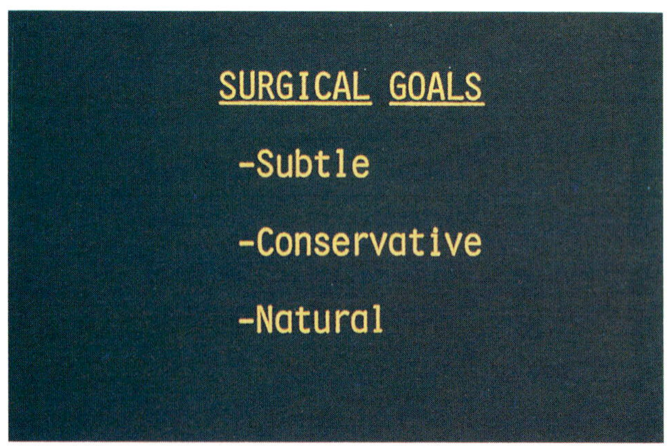

Figure 94. Effective visual presentation containing key words for emphasis.

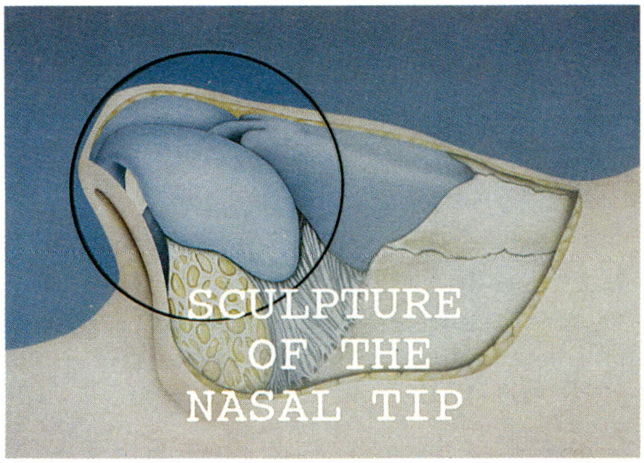

Figure 95. Word slide sandwiched over interesting background.

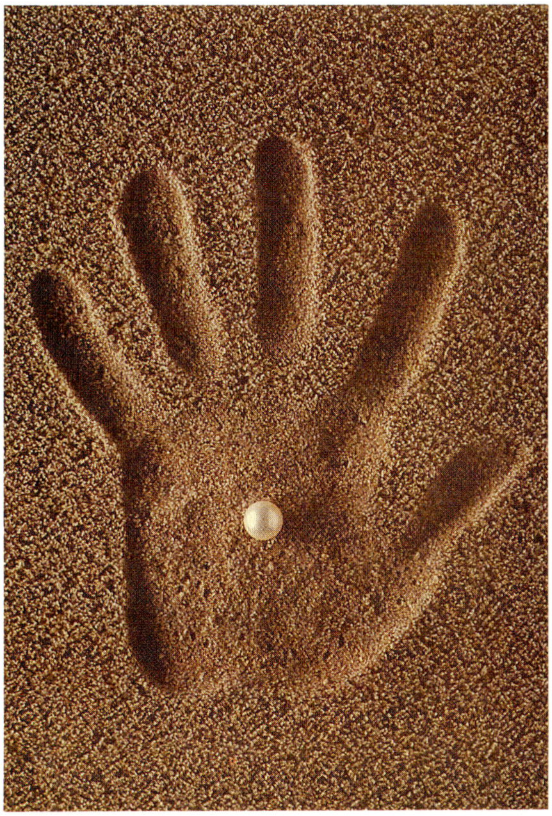

Figure 96. Initial visual image should be eye-catching and interest-provoking.

late and provoke interest and thought: "He who masters the tip, masters the nose." Short, declarative opening sentences containing strong action verbs serve best to gain immediate audience attention, stimulating curiosity about what is to follow. Lengthy introductions to the subject, particularly those that chronologically review the past history of the subject or procedure, are deadly dull and waste precious time. The printed manuscript can better accommodate historical references.

In similar fashion, the opening visual (or dual visuals) presentation is equally critical. It should be eye-catching and interest-provoking (Fig. 96). Title slides superimposed on (or sandwiched over) an interesting background that visually introduces the main topic are useful (Fig. 97). A word slide that poses a question to be addressed by the presentation can command immediate audience interest (Fig. 98). Each visual presentation should tell a story (Fig. 99), ideally communicating a complete thought, introducing a theme to follow, or completing a message begun earlier.

With audience attention now stimulated, the central theme or purpose of the presentation can be stated with a strong declarative sentence that is visually reinforced.

The effective speaker avoids lengthy historical references but gives credit to prior investigators when appropriate. In short presentations the central concepts, ideas, and interpretation of the subject at hand should be addressed, unencumbered by minute procedural details. Experimental designs and data interpretation are often best presented visually for immediate recognition and understanding. Finally, the summary and conclusion should be stated in no more than two paragraphs.

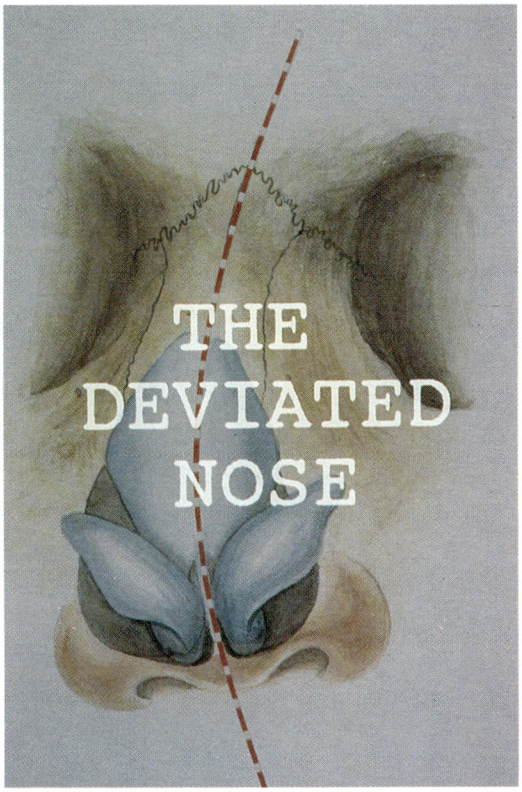

Figure 97. Initial visual slide utilizing sandwich technique.

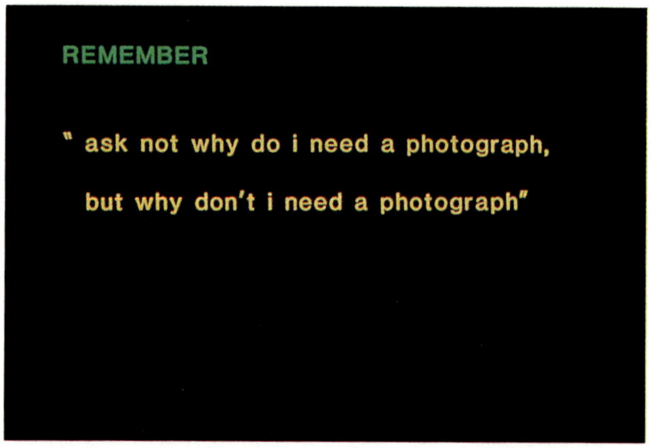

Figure 98. Initially posing a provocative question for the audience commands immediate audience interaction.

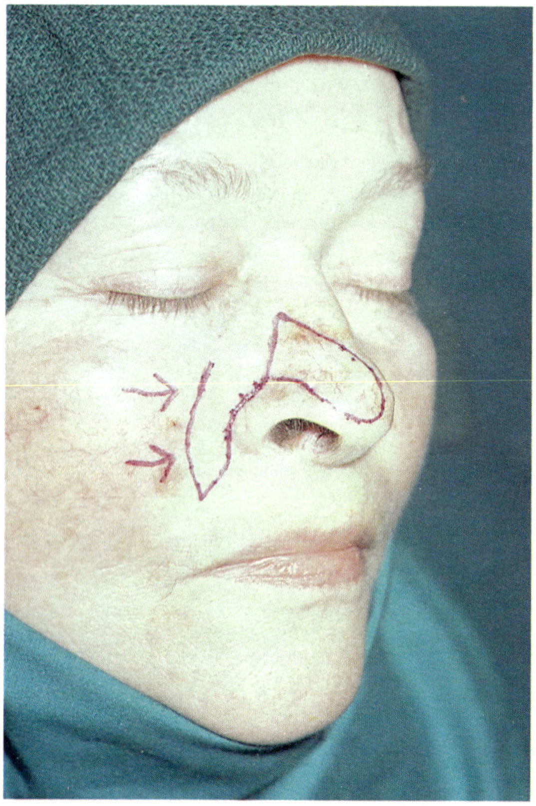

Figure 99. Visual aid that "tells a story."

DESIGN OF VISUAL AIDS

Informational word slides are most effective when an economy of words is used to convey a concept (Fig. 100a-b). Whenever possible, they should be self-explanatory; if a waivering pointer is required to describe them, they should be redesigned.

Word slides using all upper case bold letters are visually preferable to those using upper and lower case (Fig. 101a-b). The Kroy lettering machine can be put to affective use in designing letters with hard, sharp edges (Fig. 102). If an IBM typewriter is to be used, the type should be clean and with sharp edges.

In design, the word slides should not exceed eight to ten lines of type and not more than 25 characters per line (Fig. 103). A reliable rule of thumb is to hold the slide to the light and read the type. If legible to the naked eye, it will probably serve well for a large audience when projected. If not, the slide should be redesigned.

a

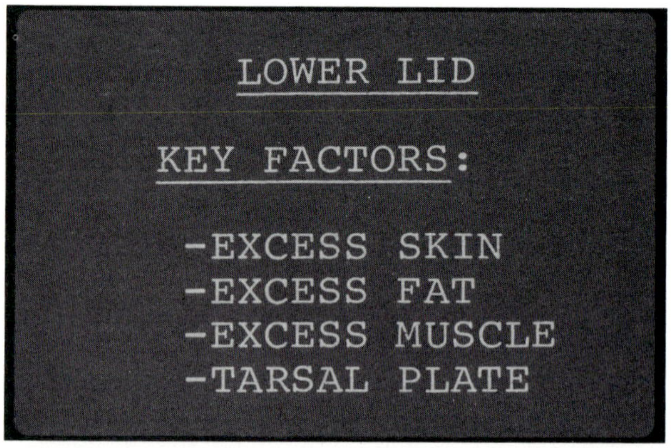

b

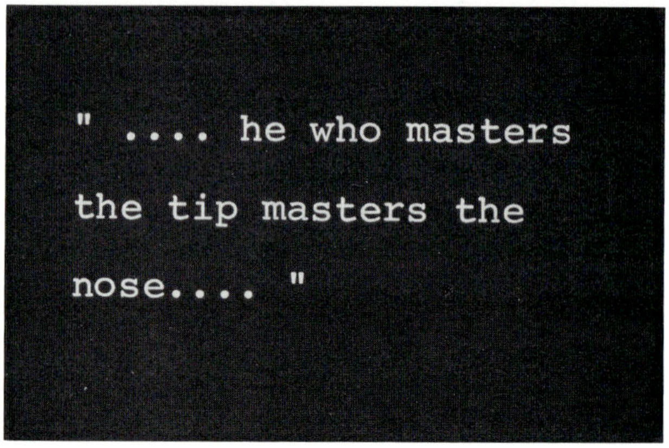

Figure 100. a,b, Word slides impart greater impact when an economy of words is used to communicate a single concept or idea.

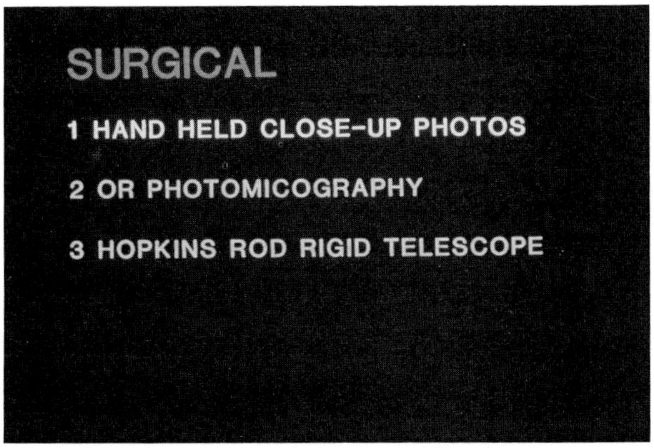

a

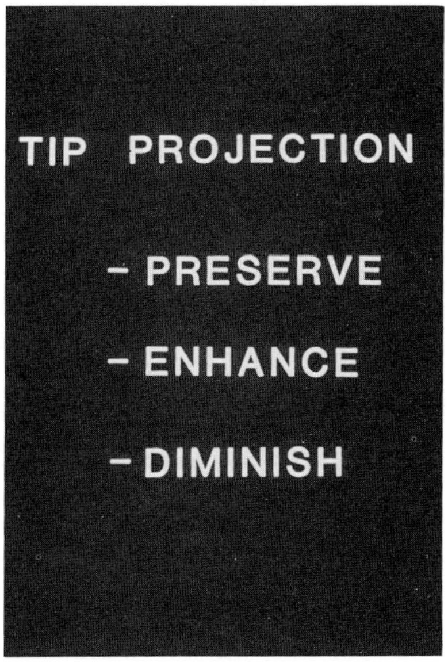

b

Figure 101. **a,b,** Upper case letters are usually best for word slides containing only a few words. If information of varying importance or emphasis is to be communicated, both upper and lower case can be appropriately used.

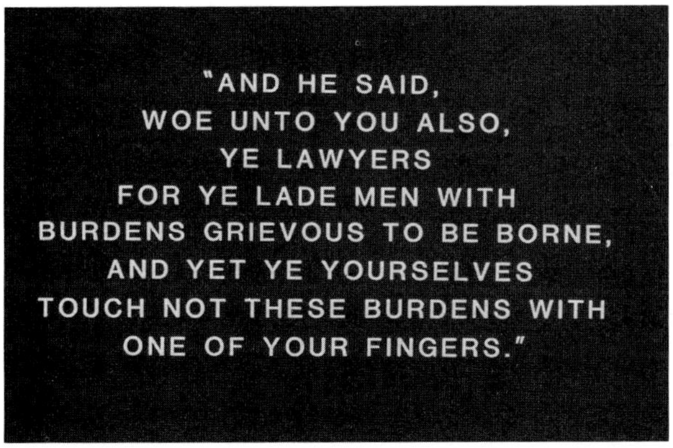

Figure 102. Word slide produced with Kroy lettering machine.

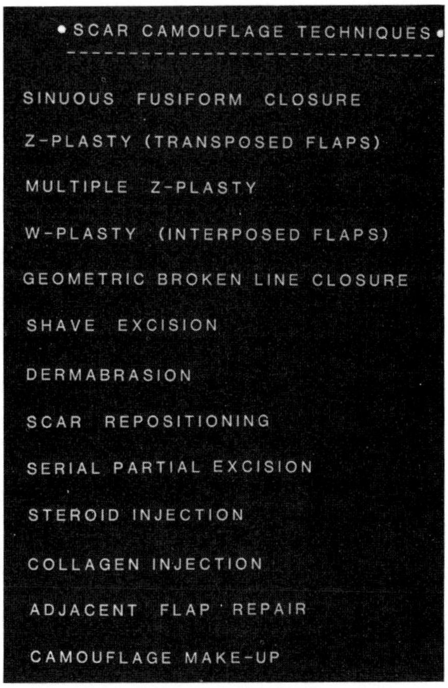

Figure 103. Word slides should contain no more than eight to ten lines of type and, in general, not more than 25 characters.

6 The Organized System

Photographic Informed Consent

Informed consent of the patient for any planned surgical procedure has become the watchword of modern medicine. So, too, must a photographic record of any area of a patient's face. This irrefutable rule becomes even more critical in facial surgery, since the opportunity for the patient to be recognized through his photograph is ever present. Although it is the right of every individual to refuse to give permission for facial photography, just as it is his right to refuse a recommended surgical treatment plan, it is rare for any patient desirous of a change in facial appearance to fail to understand the importance of the photographic record to the surgeon. (Our policy with a patient who absolutely refuses to submit to photography, despite careful explanations of the absolute requirement for recording facial characteristics for analysis and planning, is to refuse, gently but steadfastly, to carry on with the desired treatment plan. Such patients, although rare, almost always are poor candidates for image-changing surgery.)

The occasional patient who wishes to remain anonymous will consent to photography for planning and confidential record-keeping, but refuse permission for publication of the photograph or for it to be used in medical teaching situations. Although this places undue restrictions on surgical teachers in particular, it does not automatically disqualify a patient as a good candidate for surgery, since individuals in the public eye may quite appropriately require anonymity.

The vast majority clearly understand the significant need for standard and uniform pre- and postoperative photography in facial plastic surgery, particularly when they are told of the important need for accurate photographs in presurgical planning. Just as the orthopedist requires radiographs for proper fracture repair and the cardiologist depends on electrocardiograms for accurate monitoring of cardiac activity, the surgeon operating in the head and neck area relies on near-perfect facial photographs to carry out accurate surgery and to follow the postsurgical appearance carefully. When made aware of these logical medical comparisons, seldom will any reasonable patient refuse to follow the surgeon's instructions.

In our practice, patients sign a comprehensive photographic permission form on two or, often, three occasions (Fig. 104). During the first consultation in the office when the preoperative photographs are taken by the surgeon, the initial comprehensive permit form is explained and signed. Later, on admission to the hospital, a second similar hospital photographic permission form is completed. In addition, the hospital surgical operative consent includes appropriate permission for preoperative, intraoperative, and postoperative photography. For minors, of course, the signed permission for surgery as well as photography must be obtained from the appropriate parent or guardian. If for any reason a patient is unable to sign, proper verbal consent may be obtained in the presence of two witnesses.

STORAGE AND RETRIEVAL OF PHOTOGRAPHS

The finest photograph in the world is of no value if misplaced or not readily retrievable. Cross-indexing systems and computerized codings may be of extreme value in large slide collections, but the finest system will thrive or wither based on one critical variable—the *person* who identifies, catalogues, cross-indexes, labels, stores, and retrieves the photograph or slide transparency (Fig. 105). In some successful systems this individual may be the physician; more likely it is a dedicated employee or secretary.

Large university and medical centers that can assign several employees to slide storage and retrieval usually have evolved cataloguing systems specific to their needs and interests.

In private small office settings, less formal systems are the rule. One such system will be described in detail.

All 35 mm Kodachrome 25 slides of each new patient, when developed, are labeled with the patient's name which is keyed to a chronological list com-

M. EUGENE TARDY, JR., M. D.

HEAD AND NECK PLASTIC SURGERY, LTD.

2900 North Lake Shore Drive Manor Suite 430 Chicago, Illinois 60657
Phone 312/472-7559

ST. JOSEPH HOSPITAL
2900 LAKE SHORE DRIVE
CHICAGO, IL 60657
Tel. 312/975-3000

RECORD OF AUTHORIZATION FOR TAKING AND PUBLICATION OF PHOTOGRAPHS

In connection with the medical services, which I am receiving from my physician, M. Eugene Tardy, Jr., M.D., I consent that photographs may be taken of me or parts of my body, under the following conditions:

A. The photographs may be taken only with the consent of my physician and under such conditions and at such time as may be approved by him.

B. The photographs shall be taken by my physician or by a photographer approved by my physician.

C. The photographs shall be used for medical records, and if in the judgement of my attending physician, medical research, education or science will be benefited by their use, such photographs and information relating to my case may be published and republished, either separately or in connection with each other, in professional journals or medical books, or used for any other purpose which he may deem proper in the interest of medical education, knowledge, or research; provided, however, that it is specifically understood that in any such publication or use I shall not be identified by name.

Patient's Signature: ______________________

(If a minor or patient is unable to affix signature)
Authority to Sign Consent: (Type or Print)

______________________ Witness: ______________________

Signed: ______________________ Address: ______________________

Relationship: ______________________ ______________________

Address: ______________________

____

Figure 104. A typical photography consent form, agreed to and signed by the patient both in the office and on admission to the hospital.

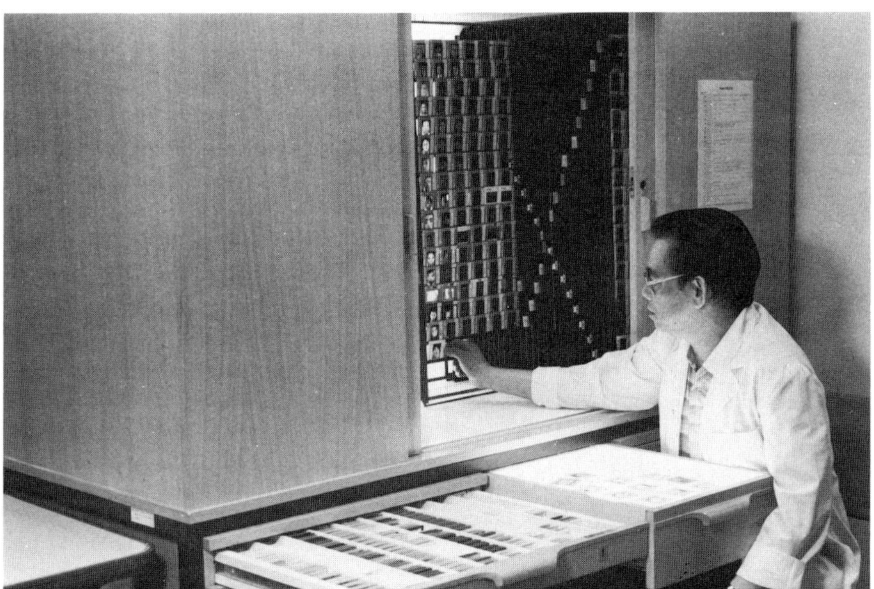

Figure 105. The single most critical link in any slide cataloguing system is the dedicated, compulsive person who stores and retrieves every slide.

piled as each patient is photographed (Fig. 106). Pertinent information is added ("Pre" if patient is preoperative, and additional information if it is judged valuable). Each of the slides is then filed alphabetically in 8½ × 11 plastic slide holders encased in manila folders bearing the patient's name (Fig. 107), and this remains undisturbed until required for patient viewing or preoperative planning. At the time of surgery, necessary views of the patient are *projected life size and in color in the operating room* for constant reference during surgery. A useful teaching tool is projection of slides on the flat surface of a Dry-Erase board. With special colored markers, incisions may be plotted, tissue correction planned, and proportions and angles illustrated (Fig. 108). Erasure is swift and easy, allowing for replanning and reillustration.

Slides of patients taken during surgery and at planned intervals after surgery can concurrently be filed consecutively in the same plastic folders, allowing quick and easy comparison of corrective changes and healing results (Fig. 109a-c). The interval after surgery is appropriately marked on each series of slides.

This system of slide storage and retrieval serves well for routine cataloguing. Further indexing and triple or quadruple cross-referencing can be employed, cross-indexing patient's name, diagnosis, and surgical procedure or procedures. Almost unlimited cross-indexing lends itself well to microcom-

Figure 107. Nonpolyvinyl chloride plastic sheets are useful in systematic storage and comparison of serial photographs.

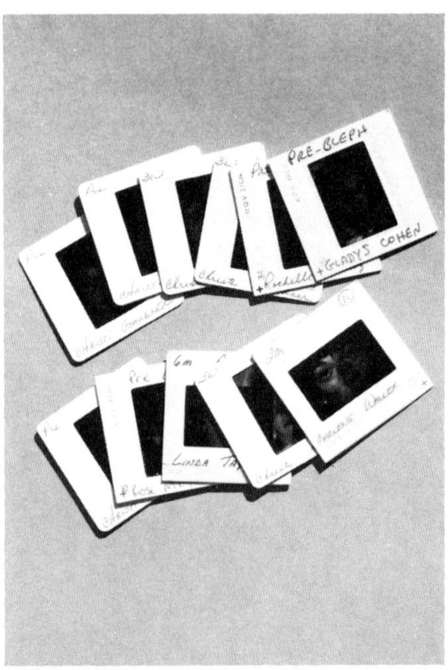

Figure 106. Upon return from processing, each slide is immediately labeled with patient name and other essential information before storage and cataloguing.

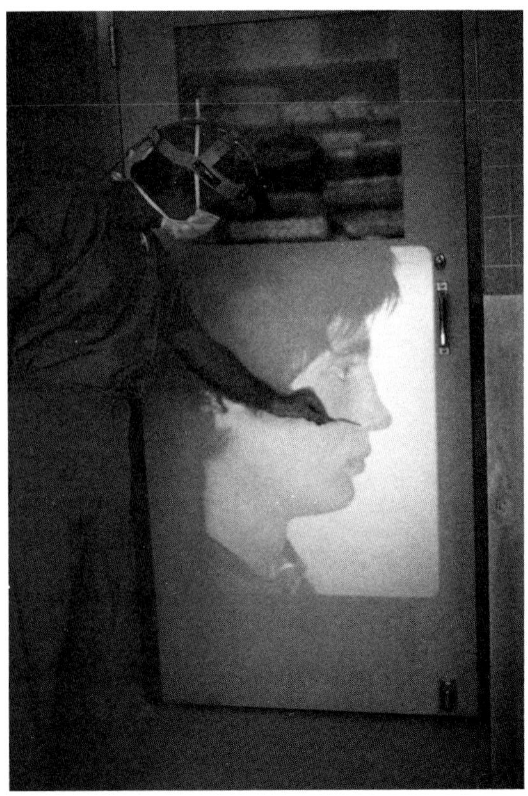

Figure 108. Patient slides are projected on a large Dry-Erase board in the operating room for easy surgical reference and facilitation of teaching. The intended operation may be rehearsed, diagrammed, and discussed as often as desired without alterating the original projected image.

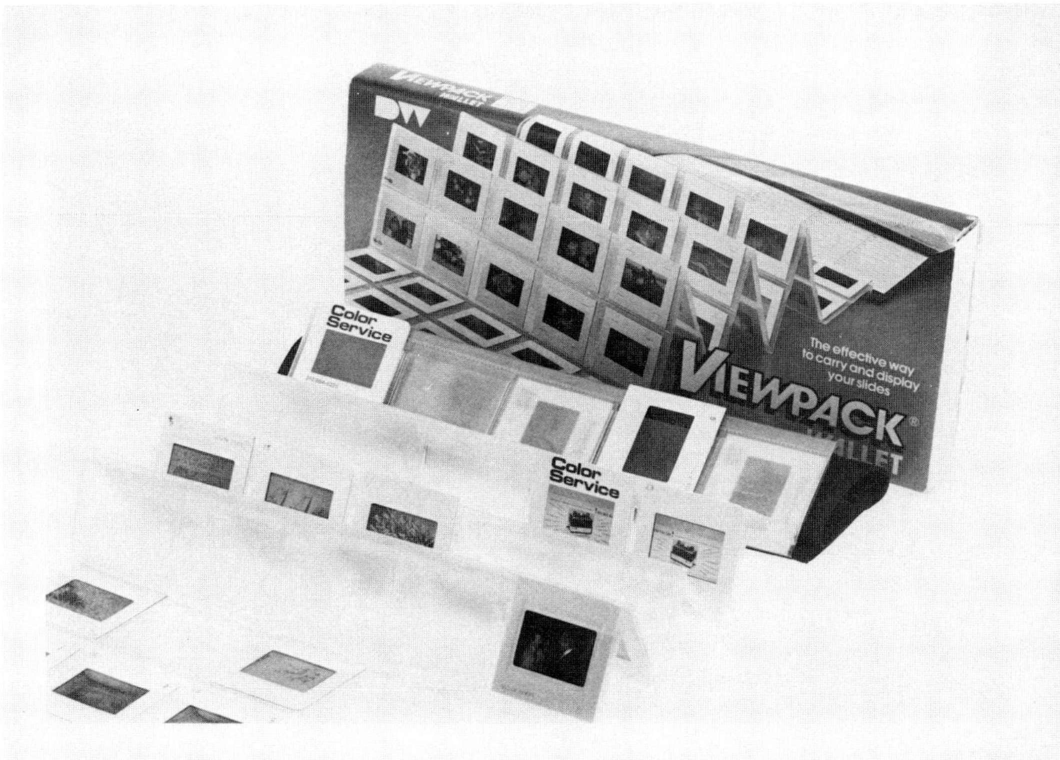

a

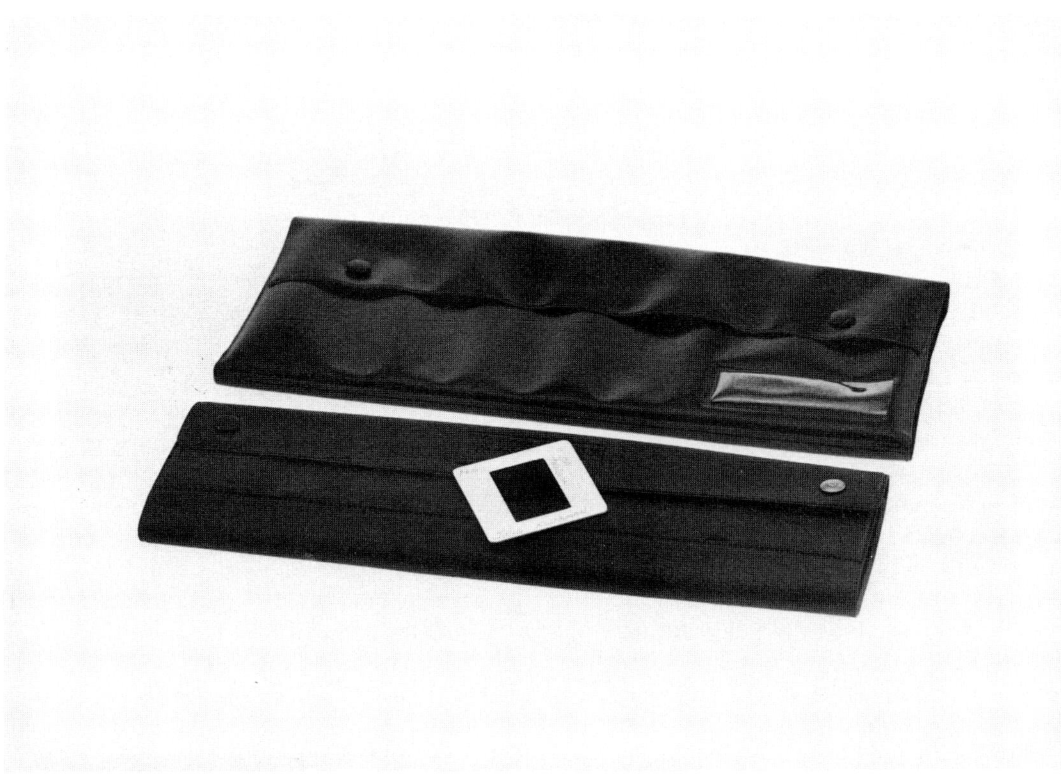

b

Figure 109. **a,** Quick serial comparison of filed 2 × 2 slides filed in plastic folders. **b,c,** Storage and easy transport of slides in slide wallets of various sizes and capacities.

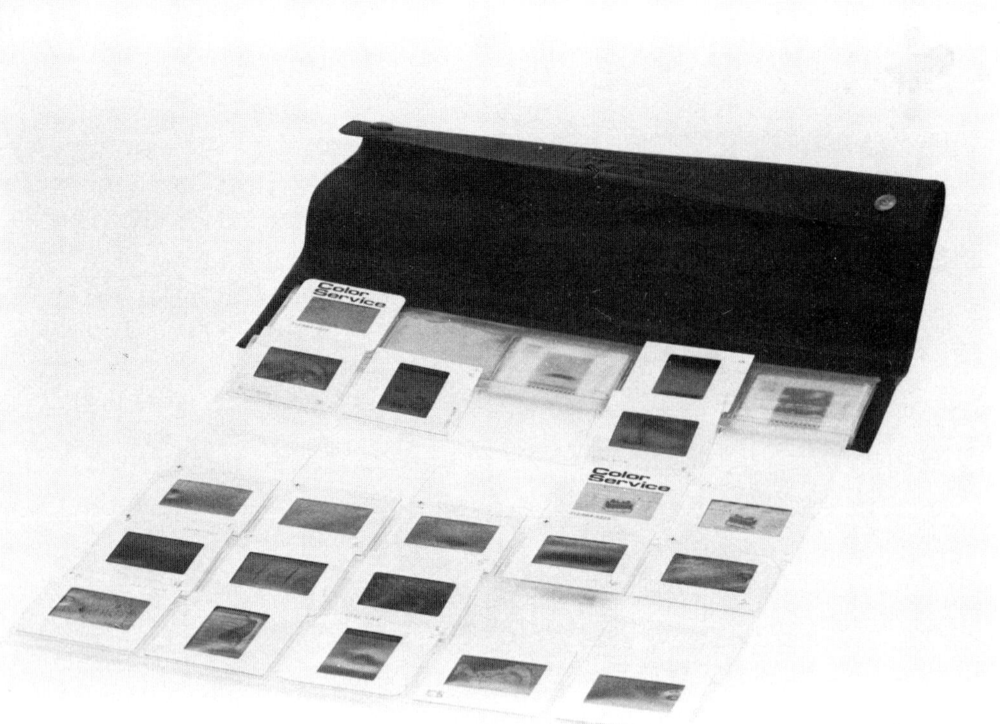

c

Figure 109. (*Continued*)

puter information storage, but still requires a *reliable* person to store and retrieve slides accurately.

A second system involves storage of slides that constitute lectures and presentations. For recurring use, the Kodak Carousel 80 slide tray, stored and labeled in the provided protective box (Fig. 110), allows convenience and easy accessibility of material frequently used ("Management of Epistaxis," "Correction of the Twisted Nose"). Although these lecture presentations are constantly being upgraded, augmented, or refined, storage in carousel trays facilitates rapid retrieval and lecture presentation. Patient slides contained in these trays are usually duplicate copies of the master slides kept in plastic sheets described in the first system, or extra master slides taken at the time the patient is photographed (a plan preferable to slide duplication).

System 3 is an extension of System 2. Transporting large numbers of slides to meetings and courses is difficult and bulky if many carousel trays are required. Metal slide box organizers solve this special problem and further protect the slide emulsions by repelling airport security check x-rays (Fig. 111a-c). Although heavy when fully laden with slides, vast numbers of slides can be transported in a limited space and kept well organized for carousel loading at the meeting. Sturdy plastic storage trays are also useful.

System 4 involves the storage of special slides, such as word slides, "joke" slides, unusual or rare conditions, and special illustrations, in large slide storage cabinets designed by Multiplex or Abodia (see Fig. 105). Here extra slides that are frequently pulled in and out for presentations may be rapidly stored and retrieved under direct vision. Rapid visualization of many slides is the major virtue of this system. Slides that fit awkwardly into any organized cataloguing system—and we all encounter them—may be quickly and conveniently filed here until further disposition is required.

It is apparent then that no single system can accommodate all storage-retrieval possibilities and contingencies. The systems described interface well and lend themselves to easy accessibility and computerized or file card cross-indexing.

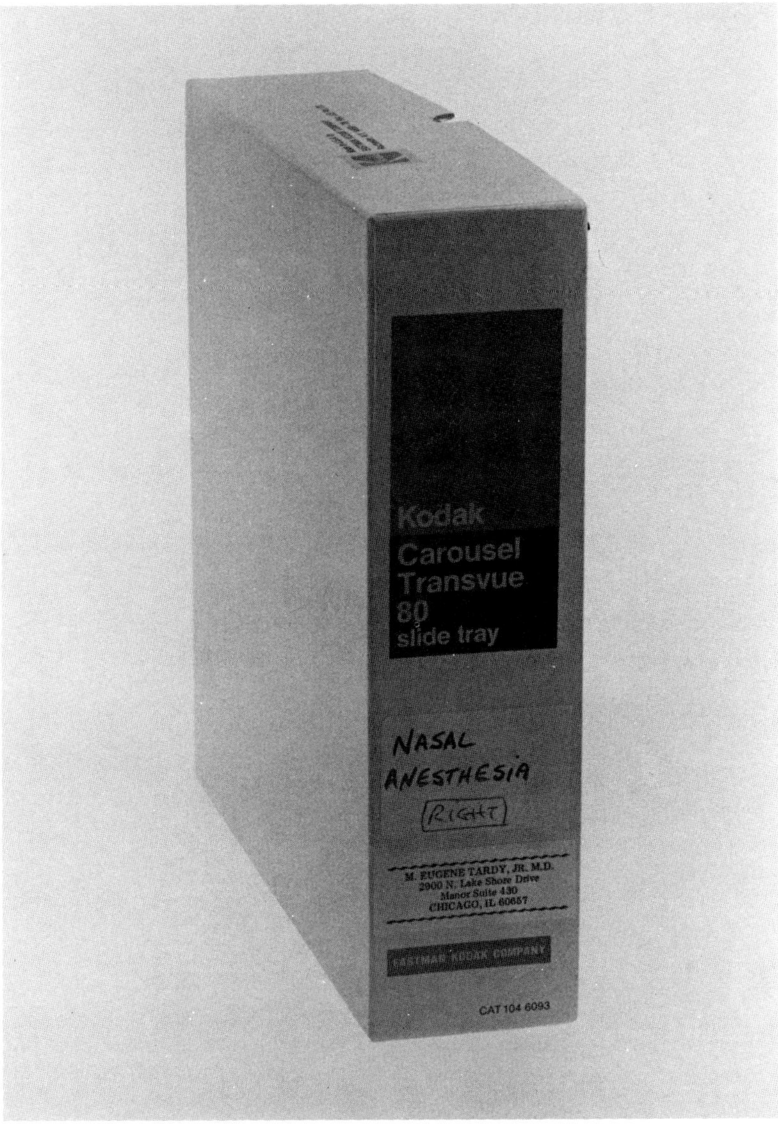

Figure 110. Standard carousel trays store 80 2 × 2 slides for more routine presentations and lectures.

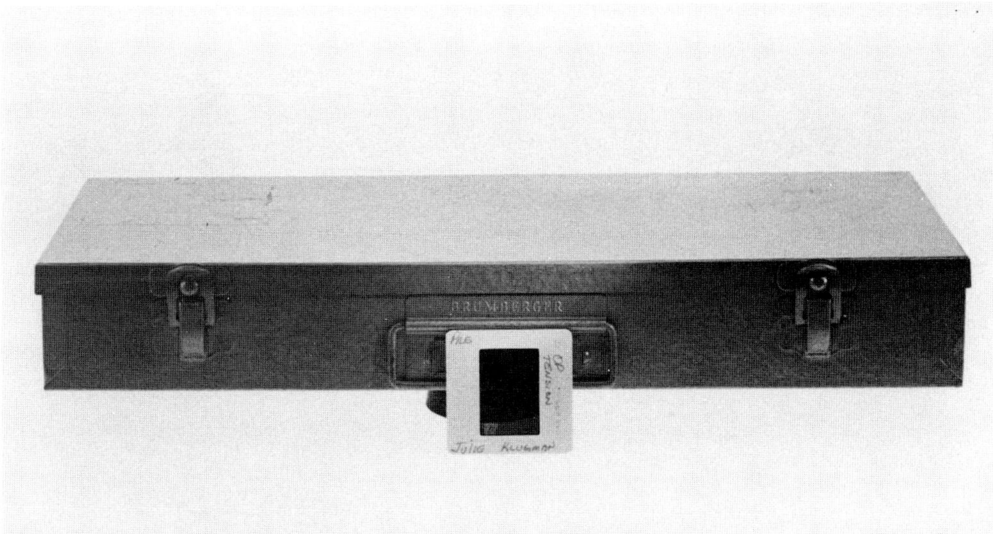

Figure 111. a,b, Metal slide trays made by Brumberger are extremely sturdy, store hundreds of slides, and protect them from the damage possible when slides are passed through airport x-ray machines scores of times. **c,** Sturdy plastic storage trays are lighter in weight but highly protective and portable.

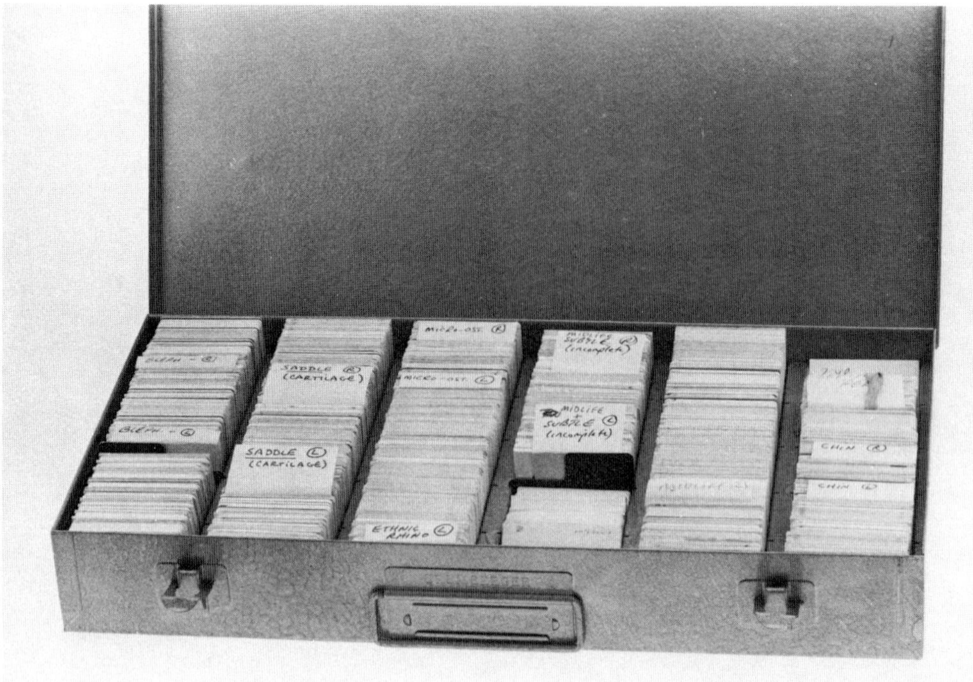

b

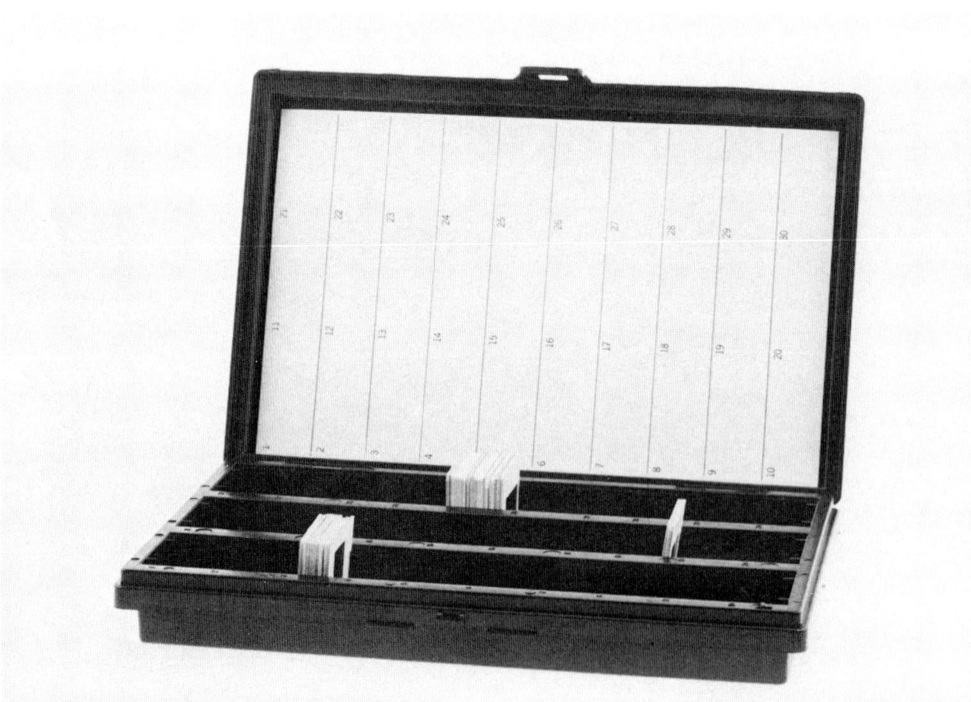

c

Figure 111. *(Continued)*

Index